whdra 12/6/23

MRI

Second Edition

MRI
BASIC PRINCIPLES AND APPLICATIONS
SECOND EDITION

Mark A. Brown, PhD
Senior Technical Instructor
Siemens Training and Development Center
Cary, NC 27511

Richard C. Semelka, MD
Professor and Director of MR Services
Department of Radiology
University of North Carolina School of Medicine
Chapel Hill, NC 27599

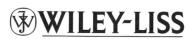WILEY-LISS

A JOHN WILEY & SONS, INC., PUBLICATION
New York • Chichester • Weinheim • Brisbane • Singapore • Toronto

For ordering and customer service, call 1-800-CALL-WILEY.

Library of Congress Cataloging-in-Publication Data:

Brown, Mark A., 1955–
    MRI : basic principles and applications / Mark Brown and Richard
C. Semelka. — 2nd ed.
        p.   cm.
    Includes bibliographical references and index.
    ISBN 0-471-33062-0 (paper : alk. paper)
    1. Magnetic resonance imaging.   I. Semelka, Richard C.
II. Title.
    [DLNM: 1. Magnetic Resonance Imaging   WN 185 B879m   1999]
RC78.7.N83B765   1999
616.07'548—dc21
DNLM/DLC   99-12462
for Library of Congress   CIP

Printed in the United States of America

10 9 8 7 6 5 4 3

◼️ CONTENTS

Our intention in writing the first edition of *MRI: Basic Principles and Applications* was to provide a book that would serve as a bridge between the theory of magnetic resonance imaging (MRI) and its implementation in commercial scanners. We minimized the use of intense mathematical formalism and attempted to stress the practical aspects of MRI as it is currently used. Our attempt was to provide a resource for those medical personnel who needed accurate and detailed information yet could not devote time to study an in-depth theoretical treatise.

In the second edition we have maintained the basic organization of the first edition. The first three chapters describe the basic principles behind magnetic resonance as they are applied in the production of image contrast. Chapters 4 through 6 describe the principles used for spatial localization of the MR signal and many of the common techniques that are commercially implemented. The next three chapters describe variations to the resulting basic techniques that increase tissue contrast or ensure the quality of the measurement. Chapters 10 through 12 illustrate some of the major applications of MRI in current use and some areas where new applications have been developed since the first edition. These include MR spectroscopy and diffusion-weighted imaging. Chapter 13 describes the major hardware components common to all MRI systems. The final chapters describe the use of contrast agents and the principles that should be considered in developing clinical protocols.

We would like to thank many people in the production of this endeavor. First, we would like to thank the technical staff at the Siemens Training and Development Center and the faculty, fellows, and staff at the University of North Carolina for their interest in this project and their assistance in its completion. We would also like to thank James R. MacFall for providing Figure 11-5. Finally, we would like to thank our families for their support and patience during the time that this manuscript was prepared.

M.A.B.
R.C.S.

In the 22 years since the first image of two capillary tubes was produced, the field of magnetic resonance imaging (MRI) has evolved into an indispensable component in the armament of imaging procedures. Much of this evolution has been accomplished through changes in localization techniques and new mechanisms of contrast. Even so, many of the fundamental principles governing image contrast and localization have changed little since they were first determined. Our purpose in writing this book is to present the basic concepts of MRI in a fashion that is comprehensible to a wide range of readers. We include equations in the text for completeness, but the general reader should not be daunted by their presence. Their understanding is not a prerequisite to understanding the accompanying text. We feel this approach will provide the reader with the tools necessary to assess the various imaging techniques and to understand and apply the contrast mechanisms inherent in each one.

This book is organized into five general sections. The first three chapters describe the source of the magnetic resonance signal and how its manipulation provides the contrast within an image. Chapters 4, 5, and 6 describe the concepts of spatial localization and various imaging techniques that are commonly used. The next four chapters describe several variations on basic imaging techniques for enhancing contrast between tissues and/or for ensuring fidelity of the detected signals. The next chapter describes the basic hardware components of any MRI system. The final chapters provide an overview of contrast agents in clinical use and clinical applications and concepts to consider in developing imaging protocols.

M.A.B.
R.C.S.

CHAPTER 1

Production of Net Magnetization

Magnetic resonance (MR) is based upon the interaction between an external magnetic field and a nucleus that possesses spin. Nuclear spin, or more precisely nuclear spin angular momentum, is one of several intrinsic characteristics of an atom and its value depends on the precise atomic composition. Every element in the periodic table except argon and cerium has at least one naturally occurring isotope that possesses spin. Thus, in principle, nearly every element can be examined using MR, and the basic ideas of resonance absorption and relaxation are common for all of these elements. The precise details will vary from element to element and from system to system.

Atoms consist of three fundamental particles: protons, which possess a positive charge; neutrons, which have no charge; and electrons, which have a negative charge. The nucleus of an atom consists of all the protons and neutrons while the electrons are located in shells or orbitals surrounding the nucleus. The characteristic properties of atoms depend upon the particular number of each of these particles. In categorizing elements, the properties most commonly used are the atomic number and the atomic weight. The *atomic number* is the number of protons in the nucleus, and is the primary index used for the delineation of atoms. All atoms of an element have the same atomic number. The *atomic weight* is the sum of the number of protons and the number of neutrons. Atoms of the same atomic number but different atomic weights are called *isotopes*.

A third property of the nucleus is spin or intrinsic spin angular momentum. The nucleus can be considered to be constantly rotating about an axis at a constant rate. This self-rotation axis is perpendicular to the direction of rotation (Figure 1-1). A limited number of values for the spin are found in nature; that is, the spin, I, is quantized to certain discrete values. These values depend on the atomic number and atomic weight of the particular nucleus. There are three groups of values for I: 0, half-integral values, and integral values. A nucleus has no spin ($I = 0$) if it has an even number atomic weight and an even atomic number.

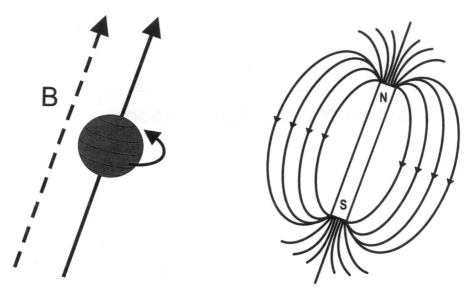

Figure 1-1. A rotating nucleus with a positive charge produces a magnetic field oriented parallel to the axis of rotation. This arrangement is analogous to a bar magnet in which the magnetic field is considered to be oriented from the south to the north pole.

Such a nucleus does not interact with an external magnetic field and cannot be studied using MR. A nucleus has an integral value for I (e.g., 1, 2, 3) if it has an even atomic weight and an odd atomic number. A nucleus has a half-integral value for I (e.g., $\frac{1}{2}$, $\frac{3}{2}$, $\frac{5}{2}$) if it has an odd atomic weight. Table 1-1 lists the spin and isotopic composition for some elements commonly found in biological systems. The ^{1}H nucleus, consisting of a single proton, is a natural choice for probing the body using MR techniques. It has a spin of $\frac{1}{2}$ and is the most abundant isotope for hydrogen. It is very sensitive to the magnetic field due to its large value for γ. Finally, the body is composed of tissues that contain primarily water and fat, both of which contain hydrogen.

Whereas an accurate mathematical description of a nucleus with spin and its interactions requires the use of quantum mechanical principles, most of MR can be described using the concepts of classical mechanics, particularly in describing the actions of a nucleus with spin. The subsequent discussions of MR phenomena in this book use a classical approach. In addition, while the concepts of resonance absorption and relaxation apply to all nuclei with spin, the description is focused on ^{1}H (commonly referred to as a proton) since most imaging experiments visualize the ^{1}H nucleus.

Table 1-1   Constants for Selected Nuclei of Biological Interest

Element	Nuclear Composition Protons	Neutrons	I	Gyromagnetic Ratio γ (MHz T^{-1})	% Natural Abundance	ω at 1.5 T (MHz)
^{1}H, Protium	1	0	1/2	42.5774	99.985	63.8646
^{2}H, Deuterium	1	1	1	6.53896	0.015	9.8036
^{3}He	2	1	1/2	32.436	0.000138	48.6540
^{12}C	6	6	0	0	98.90	0
^{13}C	6	7	1/2	10.7084	1.10	16.0621
^{14}N	7	7	1	3.07770	99.634	4.6164
^{15}N	7	8	1/2	4.3173	0.366	6.4759
^{16}O	8	8	0	0	99.762	0
^{17}O	8	9	5/2	5.7743	0.038	8.6614
^{19}F	9	10	1/2	40.0776	100	60.1164
^{23}Na	11	12	3/2	11.2686	100	16.9029
^{31}P	15	16	1/2	17.2514	100	25.8771
^{129}Xe	54	75	1/2	11.8604	26.4	17.7906

Source: Adapted from Ian Mills, ed., *Quantities, Units, and Symbols in Physical Chemistry*, IUPAC, Physical Chemistry Division, Blackwell, Oxford, UK, 1989.

   Concurrent with the spinning, positively charged nucleus (the location of the protons) is a local magnetic field or magnetic moment. This associated magnetic moment is fundamental to MR. A bar magnet provides a useful analogy. A bar magnet has a north and south pole, or more precisely, a magnitude and orientation or direction to the magnetic field can be defined. A nucleus with spin can be viewed as a vector having an axis of rotation with a definite orientation and magnitude to this axis (Figure 1-1). The associated magnetic field is parallel to the axis of rotation for the nucleus. This orientation of the nuclear spin and the changes induced due to the experimental manipulations that the nucleus undergoes provide the basis for the MR signal.

   In general, MR measurements are made on collections of similar protons rather than on an individual proton. It will prove useful to consider such a collection both as individual protons acting independently (a "microscopic" picture) and as a single entity (a "macroscopic" picture). For many concepts, the two pictures provide equivalent results, even though the microscopic picture is more complete. Conversion between the two pictures requires the principles of statistical mechanics. While necessary for a complete understanding of MR phenomenon, the nature of this conversion is beyond the scope of this book. For most concepts

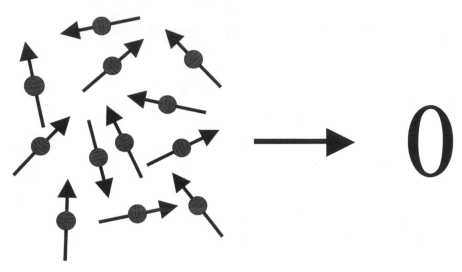

Figure 1-2. Microscopic and macroscopic pictures of a collection of protons in the absence of an external magnetic field. In the absence of a field, the protons have their spin vectors oriented randomly (microscopic picture). The vector sum of these spin vectors is zero (macroscopic picture).

presented in this book, the macroscopic picture is sufficient for an adequate description. When necessary, the microscopic picture will be used.

Consider an arbitrary volume of tissue containing protons located outside a magnetic field. Each proton has a spin vector of equal magnitude. However, the spin vectors for the entire collection of protons within the tissue are randomly oriented in all directions. Performing a vector addition of these spin vectors produces a zero sum; that is, no net magnetization is observed in the tissue (Figure 1-2).

If the tissue is placed inside a magnetic field $\mathbf{B_0}$,[1] the individual protons begin to rotate, or precess, about the magnetic field. The protons are tilted slightly away from the axis of the magnetic field, but the axis of rotation is parallel to $\mathbf{B_0}$. This precession occurs because of the interaction of the magnetic field with the moving positive charge of the nucleus. By convention, $\mathbf{B_0}$ is defined to be oriented in the z direction of a Cartesian coordinate system; the axis of precession is also the z axis. The motion of each proton can be described by a unique set of x, y (perpendicular to $\mathbf{B_0}$), and z (parallel to $\mathbf{B_0}$) coordinates. The perpen-

[1]Vector quantities with direction and magnitude are indicated by boldface type while scalar quantities that are magnitude only are indicated by regular typeface.

dicular, or transverse, coordinates are nonzero and vary with time as the proton precesses, but the z coordinate is constant with time (Figure 1-3). The rate or frequency of precession is proportional to the strength of the magnetic field and is expressed by equation [1-1], the Larmor equation:

$$\omega_0 = \gamma B_0/2\pi \qquad\qquad [1\text{-}1]$$

where ω_0 is the Larmor frequency in megahertz (MHz),[2] B_0 is the magnetic field strength in tesla (T) that the proton experiences, and γ is a constant for each nucleus in $s^{-1}\ T^{-1}$, known as the gyromagnetic ratio. Values for γ and ω at 1.5 T for several nuclei are tabulated in Table 1-1.

If a vector addition is performed, as before, for the spin vectors inside the magnetic field, the results will be slightly different than for the sum outside the field. In the direction perpendicular to B_0, the spin orientations are still randomly distributed just as they were outside the magnetic field, in spite of the time-varying nature to each transverse component. There is still no net magnetization perpendicular to B_0. However, in the direction parallel to the magnetic field, there is a different result. Because there is an orientation to the precessional axis of the proton that is constant with time, there is a constant, nonzero interaction or coupling between the proton and B_0, known as the *Zeeman interaction*. This coupling causes a difference in energy between protons aligned parallel or along B_0 and protons aligned antiparallel or against B_0. This energy difference ΔE is proportional to B_0 (Figure 1-4).

The result of the Zeeman interaction is that spins in the two orientations, parallel (also known as spin up) and antiparallel (spin down), have different energies. The orientation that is parallel to B_0 is of lower energy than the antiparallel orientation. For a collection of protons, more will be oriented parallel to B_0 than will be oriented antiparallel; that is, there is an induced polarization of the spins by the magnetic field (Figure 1-5a). The exact number of protons in each energy level is

---

[2]In many discussions of MR, ω (Greek letter omega) is used to represent angular frequency, with units of s^{-1}, while cyclical frequency, in units of Hz, is represented by ν (Greek letter nu) or f. The Larmor equation is more properly written as $\nu_0 = \gamma B_0/2\pi$. In imaging derivations, the Larmor equation is expressed as equation [1-1], using ω but with units of hertz. To minimize confusion, we follow the imaging tradition throughout this book.

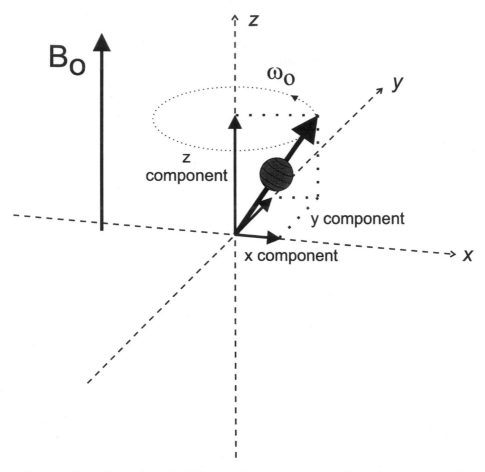

Figure 1-3. Inside a magnetic field, a proton precesses or revolves about the magnetic field. The precessional axis is parallel to the main magnetic field B_0. The z component of the spin vector (projection of the spin onto the z axis) is the component of interest because it does not change in magnitude or direction as the proton precesses. The x and y components vary with time at a frequency ω_0 proportional to B_0 as expressed by equation [1-1].

governed by a distribution known as the *Boltzmann distribution*, equation [1-2]:

$$N_{\text{UPPER}}/N_{\text{LOWER}} = e^{-\Delta E/kT} \qquad [1\text{-}2]$$

where N_{UPPER} and N_{LOWER} are the number of protons in the upper and lower energy levels, respectively, and k is Boltzmann's constant, 1.381×10^{-23} J K^{-1}. Since the separation between the energy levels ΔE de-

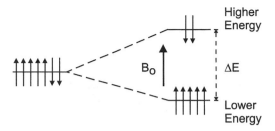

Figure 1-4. Zeeman diagram. In the absence of a magnetic field, a collection of protons will have the configurations of z components equal in energy so that there is no preferential alignment between the spin up and spin down orientations. In the presence of a magnetic field, the spin up orientation (parallel to $\mathbf{B}_0$) is of lower energy and its configuration contains more protons than the higher energy, spin down configuration. The difference in energy ΔE between the two levels is proportional to B_0.

pends on the field strength B_0, the exact number of spins in each level also depends on B_0 and increases with increasing B_0. For protons at room temperature ($\sim$293 K), there will typically be an excess of $1 : 10^6$ protons in the lower level out of the approximately 10^{25} protons within the tissue. This unequal number of protons in each energy level means that the vector sum of spins will be nonzero and will point parallel to

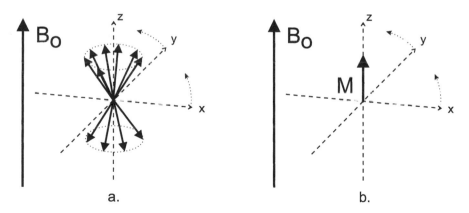

Figure 1-5. Microscopic (a) and macroscopic (b) pictures of a collection of protons in the presence of an external magnetic field. Each proton precesses about the magnetic field. If a rotating frame of reference is used with a rotation rate of ω_0, then the collection of protons appears stationary. While the z components are one of two values (one positive and one negative), the x and y components can be any value, positive or negative. The protons will appear to track along two "cones", one with a positive z component and one with a negative z component. Because there are more protons in the upper cone, there will be a nonzero vector sum $\mathbf{M}_0$, the net magnetization. It will be of constant magnitude and parallel to $\mathbf{B}_0$.

the magnetic field. In other words, the tissue will become magnetized in the presence of B_0 with a value M_0, known as the *net magnetization*; the orientation of this net magnetization will be in the same direction as B_0 and will be constant with respect to time (Figure 1-5b). This arrangement with M_0 aligned along the magnetic field with no transverse component is the normal, or equilibrium, configuration for the protons. This configuration has the lowest energy and is the arrangement to which the protons will naturally try to return following any perturbations such as energy absorption. This induced magnetization, M_0, is the source of signal for all of the MR experiments. Consequently, all other things being equal, the greater the field strength, the greater the value of M_0 and the greater the potential MR signal.

Another way to visualize this net magnetization is to recall that the individual protons are precessing about the magnetic field. When energy absorption is included, this precessional motion continues but becomes more complicated to describe. A useful technique to simplify the description is called a *rotating frame of reference*, or rotating coordinate system. In a rotating frame, the coordinate system rotates about one axis while the other two axes vary with time. By choosing a suitable axis and rate of rotation for the coordinate system, the moving object appears stationary.

For MR experiments, a convenient rotating frame uses the z axis, parallel to B_0, as the axis of rotation while the x and y axes rotate at the Larmor frequency, ω_0. When viewed in this fashion, the precessing proton appears stationary in space with a fixed set of x, y, and z coordinates. If the entire collection of protons in the tissue volume is examined, a complete range of x and y values will be found, both positive and negative, but only two z values. There will be an equal number of positive and negative x and y values, but a slight excess of positive z values, as just described. If a vector sum is performed on this collection of protons, the x and y components sum to zero but a nonzero, positive z component will be left, the net magnetization M_0. In addition, since the z axis is the axis of rotation, M_0 does not vary with time. Regardless of whether a stationary or fixed coordinate system is used, M_0 is of fixed amplitude and is parallel to the main magnetic field. For all subsequent discussions in this book, a rotating frame of reference with the rotation axis parallel to B_0 is used when describing the motion of the protons.

CHAPTER 2

Concepts of Magnetic Resonance

The MR experiment, in its most basic form, can be analyzed in terms of energy transfer. The patient or sample is exposed to energy at the correct frequency that will be absorbed. A short time later, this energy is reemitted at which time it can be detected and processed. A detailed presentation of the processes involved in this absorption and reemission are beyond the scope of this text. However, a general description of the nature of the molecular interactions is useful. In particular, the relationship between the molecular picture and the macroscopic picture provides an avenue for explanation of the principles of MR.

Chapter 1 described the formation of the net magnetization, $\mathbf{M_0}$, by the protons within a sample. The entire field of MR is based on the manipulation of $\mathbf{M_0}$. The simplest manipulation involves the application of a short burst, or pulse, of radiofrequency (rf) energy containing many frequencies. During the pulse, the protons absorb the portion of this energy at a particular frequency. Following the pulse, the protons reemit the energy at the same frequency. The particular frequency absorbed is proportional to the magnetic field B_0; the equation describing this process is the Larmor equation, equation [1-1].

The frequency of energy absorbed by an individual proton is defined very precisely by the magnetic field that the proton experiences due to the quantized nature of the spin. When a proton is irradiated with energy of the correct frequency (ω_0), it will be excited from the lower energy (spin up) orientation to the higher energy (spin down) orientation (Figure 2-1). At the same time, a proton in the higher energy level will be stimulated to release its energy and will go to the lower energy level. The energy difference (ΔE) between the two levels is exactly proportional to the frequency ω_0 and thus the magnetic field B_0:

$$\Delta E = \hbar\omega_0 = h\gamma B_0/2\pi \qquad [2\text{-}1]$$

where h is Planck's constant, 6.626×10^{-34} J s, and $\hbar$ is h divided by 2π. Only energy at this frequency stimulates transitions between the spin

9

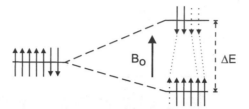

Figure 2-1. Zeeman diagram. The difference in energy ΔE between the two configurations (spin up and spin down) is proportional to the magnetic field strength B_0 and the corresponding precessional frequency ω_0 as expressed in equation [2-1]. When energy at this frequency is applied, a spin from the lower energy state is excited to the upper energy state. Also, a spin from the upper energy state is stimulated to give up its energy and relax to the lower energy state. Because there are more spins in the lower energy state, there is a net absorption of energy by the spins in the sample.

up and spin down energy levels. This quantized energy absorption is known as *resonance absorption* and the frequency of energy is known as the *resonant frequency*.

Although an individual proton absorbs the radiofrequency energy, it is more useful to discuss the resonance condition by examining the impact of the energy absorption on the net magnetization M_0. When considering a large number of protons, such as in a volume of tissue, there is a significant amount of both absorption and emission occurring during the pulse. However, because there are more protons in the lower energy level (Figure 2-1), there will be a net absorption of energy by the tissue. The energy is applied as an rf pulse with a central frequency ω_0 and an orientation perpendicular to B_0 as indicated by an effective field B_1 (Figure 2-2). This orientation difference allows a coupling between the rf pulse and M_0 so that energy can be transferred to the protons. Absorption of the rf energy of frequency ω_0 causes M_0 to rotate away from its equilibrium orientation, perpendicular to both B_0 and B_1. If the transmitter is left on long enough and at a high enough amplitude, the absorbed energy causes M_0 to rotate entirely into the transverse plane, a result known as a *90° pulse*. The direction of rotation of M_0 is perpendicular to both B_0 and B_1. When viewed in the rotating frame, the motion of M_0 is a simple vector rotation; however, the end result is the same whether a rotating or stationary frame of reference is used.

When the transmitter is turned off, the protons immediately begin to realign themselves and return to their original equilibrium orientation. They emit energy at frequency ω_0 as they do so. If a loop of wire (receiver) is placed perpendicular to the transverse plane, the protons

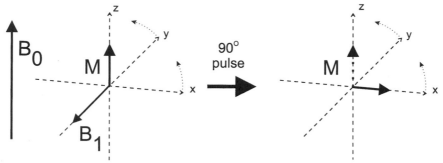

Figure 2-2. Effect of a 90° rf pulse in rotating frame of reference. The rf pulse broadcast at the resonant frequency ω_0 can be treated as an additional magnetic field $\mathbf{B}_1$ oriented perpendicular to $\mathbf{B}_0$. When energy is applied at the appropriate frequency, the protons absorb it and $\mathbf{M}$ rotates into the transverse plane. The direction of rotation is perpendicular to both $\mathbf{B}_0$ and $\mathbf{B}_1$.

induce a voltage in the wire during their precession. This voltage decays with time as more of the protons give up their absorbed energy through a process known as *relaxation* (see Chapter 3). The induced voltage, the MR signal, is known at the FID or free induction decay (Figure 2-3*a*). The magnitude of the FID signal depends on the value of $\mathbf{M}_0$ immediately prior to the 90° pulse.

In general, three aspects of an MR signal are of interest: its magnitude or amplitude, its frequency, and its phase relative to the rf transmitter phase (Figure 2-4). As mentioned previously, the signal magnitude is related to the value of $\mathbf{M}_0$ immediately prior to the rf pulse. The signal frequency is related to the magnetic field influencing the protons. If all the protons experience the same magnetic field $\mathbf{B}_0$, then only one frequency would be contained within the FID. In reality, there are many magnetic fields throughout the magnet, and thus many MR signals at many frequencies following the rf pulse. These signals are superimposed so that the FID consists of many frequencies as a function of time. It is easier to examine such a multicomponent signal in terms of frequency rather than of time. The conversion of the signal amplitudes from a function of time to a function of frequency is accomplished using a mathematical operation called the *Fourier transformation*. In the frequency presentation or frequency domain spectrum, the MR signal is mapped according to its frequency relative to the transmitter frequency ω_{TR}. For systems using quadrature detectors, ω_{TR} is centered in the display with frequencies higher and lower than ω_{TR} located to the left and right, respectively (Figure 2-3*b*). The frequency domain thus allows a

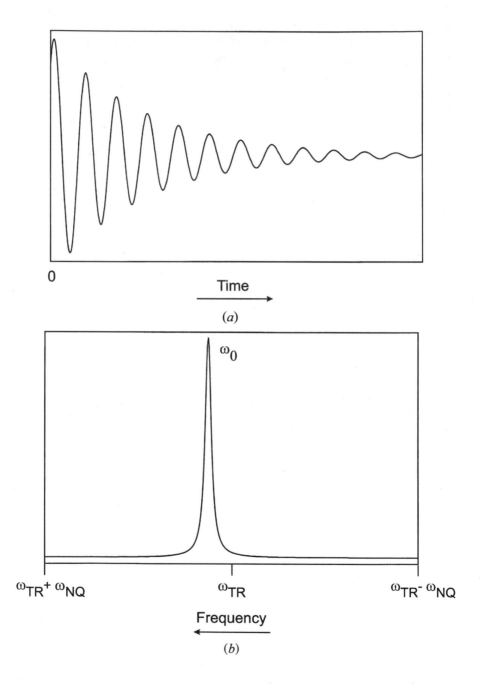

Time

(a)

ω_0

$\omega_{TR}{}^{+} \omega_{NQ}$ ω_{TR} $\omega_{TR}{}^{-} \omega_{NQ}$

Frequency

(b)

simple way to examine the magnetic environment that a proton experiences. This simplification is not without a penalty. Use of the Fourier transformation loses the ability to directly relate signal intensities to the number of protons. However, the signal intensity can be related from one frequency to another within the same measurement; that is, only relative signal intensities can be compared. Absolute signal intensities cannot be obtained without using an external reference standard.

Whereas the MR signal is analog or continuous in nature, postprocessing techniques such as Fourier transformation requires a digital representation of the signal. To produce a digital version of the signal, the FID signal is measured using an analog-to-digital converter (ADC). In most instances, the resonant frequencies of protons are greater than many ADCs can process. For this reason, a phase-coherent difference signal is generated based on the frequency and phase of the input rf pulse; that is, the signal actually digitized is the measured signal relative to ω_{TR}. Under normal conditions, this so-called demodulated signal is digitized for a predetermined time known as the *sampling time* and with a user-selectable number of data points. In such a situation, a maximum frequency, known as the *Nyquist frequency*, ω_{NQ}, can be accurately measured:

$$\omega_{NQ} = (\text{Total number of data points})/[2 * (\text{Sampling time})] \quad [2\text{-}2]$$

The Nyquist frequency in MR can be 500–500,000 Hz, depending on the combination of sampling time and number of data points. To exclude frequencies greater than the Nyquist limit prior to digitization, a filter known as a *low pass filter* is used. Frequencies excluded by the low pass filter are usually noise, so that filtering provides a method for improving the signal-to-noise ration (S/N) for the measurement. The op-

---

Figure 2-3. (*a*) Free induction decay, real part. The response of the net magnetization **M** to an rf pulse as a function of time is known as the free induction decay or FID. It is proportional to the amount of transverse magnetization generated by the pulse. The FID is maximized when using a 90° excitation pulse. (*b*) Magnitude Fourier transformation of Figure 2-3*a*. The Fourier transformation is used to convert the digital version of the MR signal (FID) from a function of time to a function of frequency. Signals measured with a quadrature detector are displayed with the transmitter (reference) frequency ω_{TR} in the middle of the display. The Nyquist frequency ω_{NQ} below and above ω_{TR} are the minimum and maximum frequencies of the frequency display, respectively. For historical reasons, frequencies are plotted with lower frequencies on the right side and higher frequencies on the left side of the display.

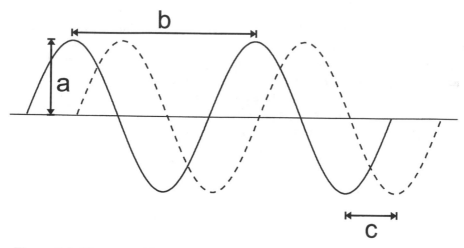

Figure 2-4. Three quantities are necessary to describe a time-varying wave. The amplitude (*a*) is the maximum deviation of the wave from its mean value. The period (*b*) is the time required for completion of one complete cycle of the wave. The frequency of the wave is the reciprocal of the period. The phase or phase angle of the wave (*c*) describes the shift in the wave relative to a reference wave. The two waves displayed have the same amplitude and period (frequency), but have a phase difference of $\pi/4$ or 90°.

timum S/N is usually obtained by increasing the sampling time to reduce the Nyquist frequency and low pass filter for the particular measurement conditions. For quadrature detection systems typically used in MR, the total receiver bandwidth is $2 * \omega_{NQ}$ centered about ω_{TR} (Figure 2-3*b*).

The specific frequency that a proton absorbs is dependent on magnetic fields arising from two sources. One is the applied magnetic field $\mathbf{B}_0$. The other one is molecular in origin and produces the chemical shift. In patients, the bulk of the MR signals arise from two sources, water and fat. Water has two hydrogen atoms bonded to one oxygen atom while fat has many hydrogen atoms bonded to a long chain carbon framework (typically 10–18 carbon atoms in length). Because of its different molecular environment, a water proton has a different local magnetic field than a fat proton. This local field difference is known as *chemical shielding* and is proportional to the main magnetic field $\mathbf{B}_0$:

$$\mathbf{B}_i = \mathbf{B}_0(1 - \sigma_i) \qquad [2\text{-}3]$$

where σ_i is the shielding term for proton i. Chemical shielding produces different resonant frequencies for fat and water protons under the influence of the same main magnetic field. Rather than analyze the frequencies in absolute terms, frequency differences are often used. A useful scale to express frequency differences is the *ppm scale*, which is the resonant frequency of the proton of interest relative to a reference frequency:

$$\omega_{i(\text{ppm})} = (\omega_{i(\text{Hz})} - \omega_{\text{ref}})/\omega_{\text{ref}} \qquad [2\text{-}4]$$

Frequency differences expressed in this form are known as *chemical shifts*. While the choice of ω_{ref} is arbitrary, it is convenient to use ω_{TR} as ω_{ref}. The primary advantage of the ppm scale is that frequency differences are independent of B_0. For fat and water, the difference in chemical shifts at all field strengths is approximately 3.5 ppm, with fat at a lower frequency. At 1.0 T, this difference is 150 Hz while at 1.5 T, it is 220 Hz (Figure 2-5).

The chemical shift difference between fat and water can be visualized in the rotating frame. A 150 Hz difference in frequency means that the fat resonance precesses slower than the water resonance by 6.7 ms per cycle (1/150 Hz). The fat resonance will align with or be in phase with the water resonance every 6.7 ms at 1.0 T. For a 1.5 T MR system, the same cycling will occur every 4.5 ms (1/220 Hz) (Figure 2-6).

The 3.5 ppm chemical shift difference mentioned previously is an approximate difference. The fat resonance signal is a composite from all the protons within the fat molecule. The particular chemical com-

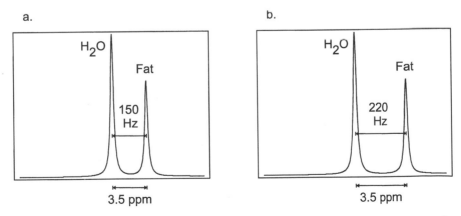

Figure 2-5. Spectrum of water and fat at 1.0 T (*a*) and 1.5 T (*b*). The resonant frequencies for water and fat are separated by approximately 3.5 ppm, which translates to an absolute frequency difference of 150 Hz for a 1.0 T magnetic field (42 MHz) or 220 Hz at a magnetic field of 1.5 T (63 MHz).

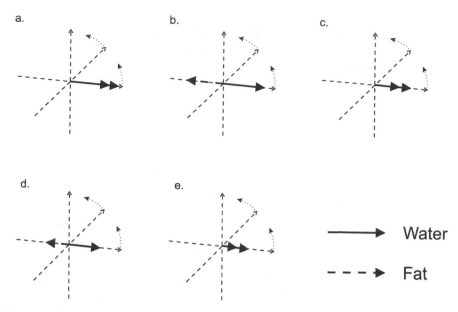

Figure 2-6. Precession of fat and water protons. Because of the 3.5 ppm frequency difference, a fat proton precesses at a slower frequency than a water proton. In a rotating frame at the water resonance frequency, the fat proton cycles in and out of phase with the water proton. Following the excitation pulse, the two protons are in phase (*a*). After a short time, they will be 180° out of phase (*b*), then in phase (*c*), then 180° out of phase (*d*), then in phase (*e*). The contribution of fat to the total signal fluctuates and depends on when the signal is detected. At 1.0 T, the in-phase times are 0 (*a*), 6.7 (*c*), and 13.3 (*e*) ms, while the out-of-phase times are 3.3 (*b*) and 10 (*e*) ms. At 1.5 T, the in-phase times are 0, 4.5, and 9 ms, while the out-of-phase times are 2.25 and 6.7 ms.

position (e.g., saturated versus unsaturated hydrocarbon chain, length of hydrocarbon chain) determines the exact resonant frequency for this composite signal. The 3.5 ppm difference applies to the majority of fatty tissues found in the body. Chemical shift differences between protons in different molecular environments provide the basis for MR spectroscopy, which is described in more detail in Chapter 12.

CHAPTER 3

Relaxation

As mentioned in Chapter 2, the MR measurement can be analyzed in terms of energy transfer. Relaxation is the process by which the protons release the energy that they absorbed from the rf pulse. Relaxation is a fundamental process in MR, as essential as energy absorption, and provides the primary mechanism for image contrast as discussed in Chapter 6. In resonance absorption, rf energy is absorbed by the protons when it is broadcast at the correct frequency. During relaxation, the protons release this energy and return to their original configuration. Although an individual proton absorbs the energy, relaxation times are measured for an entire sample and are statistical or average measurements. Relaxation times are measured for gray matter or cerebrospinal fluid as bulk samples rather than for the individual water or fat molecules within the organs. Two relaxation times can be measured, known as *T1* and *T2*. While both times measure the spontaneous energy transfer by an excited proton, they differ in the final disposition of the energy.

3.1 T1 RELAXATION AND SATURATION

The relaxation time T1 is the time required for the z component of **M** to return to 63% of its original value following an excitation pulse. It is also known as the *spin-lattice relaxation time* or *longitudinal relaxation time*. Recall from Chapter 2 that M_0 is parallel to B_0 at equilibrium and that energy absorption will rotate M_0 into the transverse plane. T1 relaxation provides the mechanism by which the protons give up their energy to return to their original orientation. If a 90° pulse is applied to a sample, M_0 will rotate as illustrated in Figure 2-2, and there will be no longitudinal magnetization following the pulse. As time goes on, a return of the longitudinal magnetization will be observed as the protons release their energy (Figure 3-1). This return of magnetization follows

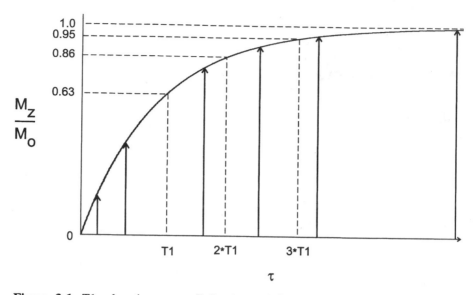

Figure 3-1. T1 relaxation curve. Following a 90° rf pulse, there is no longitudinal magnetization. A short time later, longitudinal magnetization will be observed as the protons release their energy through T1 relaxation. Gradually, as more protons release their energy, a larger fraction of M_z is reestablished. Eventually, $\mathbf{M_0}$ will be restored completely. The change of M_z/M_0 with time τ follows an exponential growth process as described by equation [3-1]. The time constant for this is T1, the spin-lattice relaxation time, and is the time when M_z has returned to 63% of its original value.

an exponential growth process, with T1 being the time constant describing the rate of growth:

$$\mathbf{M}(\tau) = \mathbf{M_0}(1 - e^{-\tau/T1}) \qquad [3\text{-}1]$$

where τ is the time following the rf pulse. After 3 T1 time periods, $\mathbf{M}$ will have returned to 95% of its value prior to the excitation pulse, $\mathbf{M_0}$. The term *spin-lattice* refers to the fact that the excited proton ("spin") transfers its energy to its surroundings ("lattice") rather than to another spin. The energy no longer contributes to spin excitation.

This energy transfer to the surroundings has some very important consequences. Suppose the rf energy is continuously applied at the resonant frequency so that no relaxation occurs. A comparison of the microscopic and macroscopic pictures is useful at this point. In the microscopic picture, the protons in the lower energy level absorb the rf energy, and the protons in the upper energy level are stimulated to emit their energy. Since energy is continuously transmitted, the proton populations of the two levels will gradually equalize. When this occurs, no further net absorption of energy is possible, a situation known as *saturation*. In the macroscopic picture, **M** will rotate continuously but gradually get smaller in magnitude until it disappears as the net population difference approaches zero. Since there is no net magnetization, there will be no coherence in the transverse plane and thus no signal is produced. This condition is known as saturation. There is a limited amount of energy that a collection of protons can absorb before they become saturated.

In a modern MR experiment, pulsed rf energy is used with a delay time between repeated pulses. This time between pulses allows the excited protons to give up the absorbed energy (T1 relaxation). As the protons give up this energy to their surroundings, the population difference (spin up versus spin down) is reestablished so that net absorption can reoccur after the next pulse. In the macroscopic picture, **M** returns toward its initial value **M₀** as more energy is dissipated. Since **M** is the ultimate source of the MR signal, the more energy dissipated, the more signal is generated following the next rf pulse.

For practical reasons, the time between successive rf pulses is usually insufficient for complete T1 relaxation so that **M** will not be completely restored to **M₀**. Application of a second rf pulse prior to complete relaxation will rotate **M** into the transverse plane, but with a smaller magnitude than following the first rf pulse. The following experiment describes the situation:

1. A 90° rf pulse is applied. **M** is rotated into the transverse plane.
2. A time τ elapses, insufficient for complete T1 relaxation. The longitudinal magnetization at the end of τ, **M'**, is less than in step 1.
3. A second 90° rf pulse is applied. **M'** is rotated into the transverse plane.
4. After a second time τ elapses, **M''** is produced. It is smaller in magnitude than **M'**, but the difference is less than the difference between **M** and **M'** (Figure 3-2).

Following a few repetitions, **M** returns to the same magnitude prior to each rf pulse; i.e., **M** achieves a steady state value. In general, this steady state value depends on five parameters: the main magnetic field **B₀**, the number of protons producing **M** (per unit volume of tissue, known as the *proton density*), the amount of energy absorbed by the protons (the pulse angle), the rate of rf pulse application (time τ), and how efficiently the protons give up their energy (T1 relaxation time). For many MRI experiments such as standard spin echo and gradient echo imaging, a steady state of **M** is present because multiple rf pulses

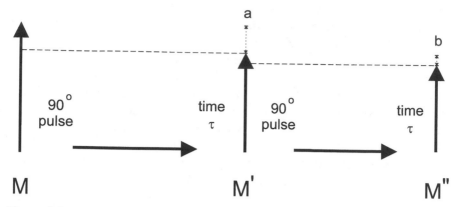

Figure 3-2. Following a 90° rf pulse, longitudinal magnetization is regenerated via T1 relaxation. If the time between successive rf pulses, τ, is insufficient for complete recovery of **M**, then only **M'** will be present at the time of the next rf pulse (*a*). If time τ elapses again, then only **M''** will be present (*b*). **M''** will be smaller than **M'**, but the difference will be less than the difference between **M** and **M'**.

are applied and the repetition time *TR* is nearly always less than sufficient for complete relaxation. To produce this steady state prior to data collection, additional rf pulses are applied to the tissue immediately prior to the main imaging pulses. These extra rf pulses are known as *preparatory pulses* or *dummy pulses* because the generated signals are usually ignored. These preparatory pulses ensure that **M** has the same magnitude prior to every measurement during the scan.

As mentioned earlier, spin-lattice relaxation measures energy transfer from an excited proton to its surroundings. The key to this energy transfer is the presence of some type of molecular motion (e.g., vibration, rotation) in the vicinity of the excited proton with an intrinsic frequency, ω_L, that matches the resonant frequency, ω_0. The closer ω_0 is to ω_L, the more readily the motion absorbs the energy and the more frequently this energy transfer occurs, allowing the collection of protons to return to its equilibrium configuration sooner. In tissues, the nature of the protein molecular structure and any metal ions that may be present have a pronounced effect on the particular ω_L. Metals ions such as iron or manganese can have significant magnetic moments that may influence the local environment. While the particular protein structures are different for many tissues, the molecular rotation or tumbling of most proteins typically have ω_L approximately 1 MHz. Therefore, at lower resonant frequencies (lower B_0), there is a better match between ω_L and ω_0. A more efficient energy transfer occurs and thus T1 is shorter. This is the basis for the frequency dependence of T1, namely, that T1 decreases with decreasing strength of the magnetic field.

3.2 T2 RELAXATION, T2* RELAXATION, AND SPIN ECHOES

The relaxation time T2 is the time required for the transverse component of $\mathbf{M}$ to decay to 37% of its initial value via irreversible processes. It is also known as the *spin-spin relaxation time* or *transverse relaxation time*. Recall from Chapter 1 that $\mathbf{M_0}$ is oriented only along the z ($\mathbf{B_0}$) axis at equilibrium and that no portion of $\mathbf{M_0}$ is in the xy plane. The coherence or uniformity of the protons is entirely longitudinal. Absorption of energy from a 90° rf pulse as in Figure 2-2 causes $\mathbf{M_0}$ to rotate entirely into the xy plane, so that the coherence is in the transverse plane at the end of the pulse. As time elapses, this coherence disappears while at the same time the protons release their energy and reorient themselves along $\mathbf{B_0}$. This disappearing coherence produces the FID described in Chapter 2. As this coherence disappears, the value of $\mathbf{M}$ in the xy plane decreases toward 0. T2 or T2* relaxation is the process by which this transverse magnetization is lost.

A comparison of the microscopic and macroscopic pictures provides additional insight. At the end of the 90° rf pulse, when the protons have absorbed energy and are oriented in the transverse plane, each proton precesses at the same frequency ω_0 and is synchronized at the same point or phase of its precessional cycle. Since a nearby proton of the same type will have the same molecular environment and the same ω_0, it can readily absorb the energy that is being released. Spin-spin relaxation refers to this energy transfer from an excited proton to another nearby proton. The absorbed energy remains as spin excitation rather than being transferred to the surroundings as in T1 relaxation. This proton–proton energy transfer can occur many times as long as the protons are in close proximity and remain at the same ω_0. Intermolecular and intramolecular interactions such as vibrations or rotations cause ω_0 to fluctuate. This fluctuation produces a gradual, irreversible loss of phase coherence to the spins as they exchange the energy and reduce the magnitude of the transverse magnetization (Figure 3-3). T2 is the time when the transverse magnetization is 37% of its value immediately after the 90° pulse when this irreversible process is the only cause for the loss of coherence. As more time elapses, this transverse coherence completely disappears, only to reform in the longitudinal direction as

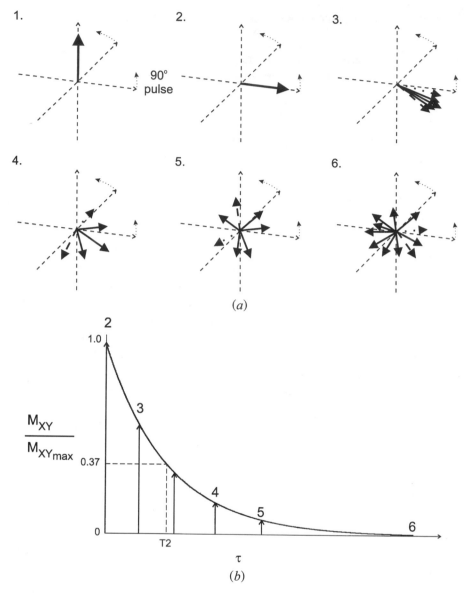

Figure 3-3. (*a*) A rotating frame slower than ω_0 is assumed for this figure. Net magnetization **M** (arrow) is oriented parallel to $\mathbf{B}_0$ (not shown) prior to pulse (1). Following a 90° rf pulse, the protons initially precess in phase in the transverse plane (2). Due to inter- and intramolecular interactions, the protons begin to precess at different frequencies (dashed arrow = faster; dotted arrow = slower) and become asynchronous with each other (3). As more time elapses (4,5), the transverse coherence becomes smaller until there is complete randomness of the transverse components and no coherence (6). (*b*) Plot of relative $\mathbf{M_{XY}}$ component. The numbers correspond to the expected $\mathbf{M_{XY}}$ component from Figure 3-3*a*. The change in $\mathbf{M_{XY}}/\mathbf{M_{XYmax}}$ with time follows an exponential decay process as described by equation [3-3]. The time constant for this process is the spin-spin relaxation time T2 and is the time when $\mathbf{M_{XY}}$ has decayed to 37% of its original value.

T1 relaxation occurs. This dephasing time T2 is always less than or equal to T1.

There are several potential causes for a loss of transverse coherence to **M**. One is the movement of the adjacent spins due to molecular vibrations or rotations. This movement is responsible for spin-spin relaxation or the true T2. Another cause arises from the fact that a proton never experiences a magnetic field that is 100% uniform or homogeneous. As the proton precesses, it experiences a fluctuating local magnetic field, causing a change in ω_0 and a loss in transverse phase coherence. This nonuniformity in $\mathbf{B}_0$ comes from three sources:

1. Main field inhomogeneity. There is always some degree of nonuniformity to $\mathbf{B}_0$ due to imperfections in magnet manufacturing, composition of nearby building walls, or other sources of metal. This field distortion is constant during the measurement time.
2. Sample-induced inhomogeneity. Differences in the magnetic susceptibility or degree of magnetic polarization of adjacent tissues (e.g., bone, air) will distort the local magnetic field near the interface between the different tissues. This inhomogeneity is of constant magnitude and is present as long as the patient is present within the magnet.
3. Imaging gradients. As discussed in Chapter 4, the technique used for spatial localization generates a magnetic field inhomogeneity that induces proton dephasing. This inhomogeneity is transient during the measurement.

Proper design of the pulse sequence eliminates the imaging gradients as a source of dephasing. The other sources contribute to the total transverse relaxation time, T2*:

$$1/T2* = 1/T2 + 1/T2_M + 1/T2_{MS} \qquad [3\text{-}2]$$

where $T2_M$ is the dephasing time due to the main field inhomogeneity and $T2_{MS}$ is the dephasing time due to the magnetic susceptibility differences. The decay of the transverse magnetization following a 90° rf pulse, the FID, follows an exponential process with the time constant of T2* rather than just T2:

$$\mathbf{M_{XY}}(\tau) = \mathbf{M_{XYmax}}\, e^{-\tau/T2*} \qquad [3\text{-}3]$$

where $\mathbf{M_{XYmax}}$ is the transverse magnetization $\mathbf{M_{XY}}$ immediately following the excitation pulse. For most tissues or liquids, $T2_M$ is the major factor in determining $T2^*$, while for tissue with significant iron deposits or air-filled cavities, $T2_{MS}$ predominates $T2^*$.

Some sources of proton dephasing can be reversed by the application of a 180° rf pulse, which is described by the following sequence of events (Figure 3-4):

1. A 90° rf pulse
2. A short delay of time τ
3. A 180° rf pulse
4. A second time delay τ

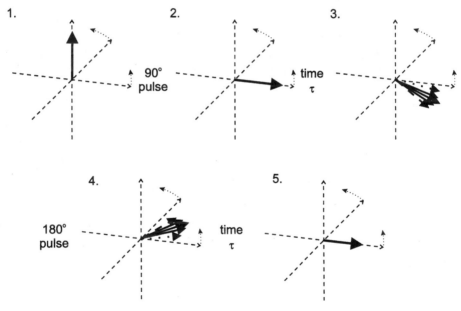

Figure 3-4. A rotation frame slower than ω_0 is assumed for this figure. Net magnetization **M** (arrow) is oriented parallel to B_0 (not shown) prior to pulse (1). Application of a 90° rf pulse rotates M_0 into the transverse plane (2). Due to $T2^*$ relaxation processes, the protons become asynchronous with each other during time τ (3). Application of a 180° rf pulse causes the protons to reverse their phase relative to the transmitter phase. The protons that precessed most rapidly are farthest behind (dashed arrow) while the slowest protons are in front (dotted arrow) (4). Allowing time τ to elapse again allows the protons to regain their phase coherence in the transverse plane (5), generating a signal in the receiver coil known as a *spin echo*. The loss in magnitude of the reformed coherence relative to the original coherence (2) is due to irreversible processes (i.e., true spin-spin or $T2$ relaxation).

The initial 90° rf pulse rotates M_0 into the transverse plane. During the time τ, proton dephasing will occur through T2* relaxation processes. Application of the 180° rf pulse causes the protons to reverse their phases relative to the resonant frequency. The rates and directions of precession for the protons do not change, only their relative phase. If time τ elapses again, then the protons will regain their transverse coherence. This reformation of phase coherence induces another signal in the receiver coil, known as a *spin echo*. Sources of dephasing that do not change during the two time periods, the main field inhomogeneity and magnetic susceptibility differences, are eliminated because the protons experience exactly the same interactions each time. This means that the contributions to T2* relaxation from these static sources will disappear. Only the irreversible spin-spin relaxation is unaffected by the 180° rf pulse so that the loss of phase coherence and signal amplitude for a spin echo is due only to true T2 relaxation.

Following the echo formation, the protons continue to precess and dephase a second time as the sources of dephasing continue to affect them. Application of a second 180° rf pulse again reverses the proton phases and generates another coherence to the protons, producing another spin echo. This second echo differs from the first echo by the increased amount of T2 relaxation contributing to the signal loss. This process of spin echo formation by 180° rf pulses can be repeated as many times as desired, until T2 relaxation completely dephases the protons. The use of multiple 180° pulses maintains phase coherence to the protons longer than the use of a single 180° rf pulse because of the significant dephasing that the field inhomogeneity induces over very short time periods.

CHAPTER 4

Principles of Magnetic Resonance Imaging

Chapter 2 described the relationship between the frequency of energy that a proton absorbs and the magnetic field strength that it experiences. The technique of magnetic resonance imaging (MRI) uses this field dependence to localize these proton frequencies to different regions of space. The magnetic field is made spatially dependent through the application of magnetic field gradients. These gradients are small perturbations to the main magnetic field $\mathbf{B}_0$ that are linearly dependent on their position within the magnet, with a typical imaging gradient producing a total field distortion of less than 1%. They are applied for short periods of time and are referred to as gradient pulses. Three physical gradients are used in imaging, one in each of the x, y, and z directions. Each one is assigned, through the operating software, to one or more of the three "logical" or functional gradients required to obtain an image: slice selection, readout or frequency encoding, and phase encoding. The particular pairing of physical and logical gradients is somewhat arbitrary and depends on the acquisition parameters and patient positioning as well as the particular manufacturer's choice of physical directions. The combination of gradient pulses, rf pulses, data sampling periods, and the timing between each of them that are used to acquire an image is known as a *pulse sequence*.

The presence of magnetic field gradients requires an expanded version of the Larmor equation given in equation [1-1]:

$$\omega_i = \gamma(\mathbf{B}_0 + \mathbf{G}\cdot\mathbf{r}_i) \qquad [4\text{-}1]$$

where ω_i is the frequency of the proton at position $\mathbf{r}_i$ and $\mathbf{G}$ is a vector representing the total gradient amplitude and direction. The dimensions of $\mathbf{G}$ are usually expressed in millitesla per meter ($mT\ m^{-1}$) or gauss per centimeter ($G\ cm^{-1}$), where $10\ mT\ m^{-1} = 1\ G\ cm^{-1}$. Equation [4-1] states that, in the presence of a gradient field, each proton will resonate at a unique frequency that depends on its exact position within the gradient field. The MR image is simply a frequency and phase map

27

of the protons generated by unique magnetic fields at each point through-out the image. The picture element, or *pixel*, intensity is proportional to the number of protons contained within the volume element, or *voxel*, weighted by the T1 and T2 relaxation times for the tissues within the voxel.

4.1   SLICE SELECTION

The initial step in MRI is the localization of the rf excitation to a region of space, which is accomplished through the use of frequency-selective excitation in conjunction with a gradient known as the slice selection gradient, G_{SS}. A frequency-selective rf pulse has two parts associated with it, a central frequency and a narrow range or bandwidth of fre-quencies (typically 1–2 kHz) (see Section 4.6 for a more detailed de-scription of selective pulses). When such a pulse is broadcast in the presence of the slice selection gradient, a narrow region of tissue achieves the resonance condition (equation [4-1]) and absorbs the rf energy. The duration of the rf pulse and its amplitude determines the amount of proton rotation (e.g., 90°, 180°). The central frequency of the pulse determines the particular location excited by the pulse when the slice selection gradient is present. Different slice positions are achieved by changing the central frequency.

The slice selection gradient amplitude determines both the slice thick-ness and slice position, regardless of the orientation. The slice thickness is determined by the bandwidth of frequencies $\Delta\omega_{SS}$ incorporated into the rf pulse:

$$\Delta\omega = \gamma\Delta(G_{SS} * \text{Thickness}) \qquad [4\text{-}2]$$

Typically, $\Delta\omega$ is fixed so that the slice thickness is changed by modifying the amplitude of G_{SS}. Thinner slices require larger G_{SS}. Once G_{SS} is determined by the slice thickness, the central frequency is calculated using equation [4-1] to bring the desired location into resonance. Mul-tislice imaging, the most commonly used approach for MRI, uses the same G_{SS} for each slice but a unique rf pulse during excitation. Each rf pulse has the same bandwidth but a different central frequency, thereby exciting a different region of tissue (Figure 4-1).

The slice orientation is determined by the particular physical gradient defined as the logical slice selection gradient. The gradient orientation is always perpendicular to the plane of the slice, so that every proton within the slice experiences the same gradient field regardless of its

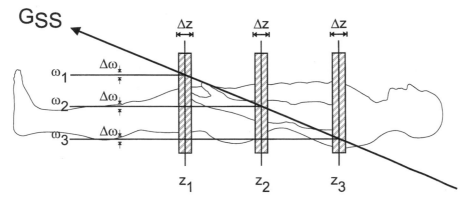

Figure 4-1. Slice selection process. In the presence of a gradient (G_{SS}), the total magnetic field that a proton experiences and the resulting resonant frequency depend on its position, according to equation [4-1]. Tissue located at position z_i will absorb rf energy broadcast with a center frequency ω_i. Each position will have a unique resonant frequency. The slice thickness Δz is determined by the amplitude of G_{SS} and by the bandwidth of transmitted frequencies $\Delta\omega_{SS}$.

position within the slice. Orthogonal slices are those in which only the *x*, *y*, or *z* gradient is used as the slice selection gradient. Oblique slices, those not in one of the principal directions, are obtained by having more than one physical gradient present when the rf pulse is broadcast. The total gradient amplitude, whether from one, two, or three physical gradients, determines the slice thickness as shown in equation [4-2]. When images are viewed on the monitor or film, the slice selection direction is always perpendicular to the surface.

4.2   READOUT OR FREQUENCY ENCODING

The readout or frequency encoding process differentiates MRI from MR spectroscopy, the other type of MR experiment (see Chapter 12). In an imaging pulse sequence, the MR signal is always detected in the presence of a gradient known as the *readout gradient*, which produces one of the two visual dimensions of the image on the film. A typical pulse sequence uses some form of excitation, such as a 90° slice selective pulse, to excite a particular region of tissue. Following excitation, the net magnetization within the slice is oriented transverse to $\mathbf{B}_0$ and will precess with frequency ω_0. T2* processes induce dephasing of this transverse magnetization (Chapter 3). This dephasing can be partially reversed to form an echo by the application of a 180° rf pulse, a gradient pulse, or both. As the echo is forming, the readout gradient $\mathbf{G}_{RO}$ is applied perpendicular to the slice direction. Under the influence of this new gradient field, the protons begin to precess at different frequencies depending on their position within it, in accordance with equation [4-1]. Each of these frequencies is superimposed into the echo. At the desired time, the echo signal is measured by the receiver coil and digitized for later Fourier transformation. The magnitude of $\mathbf{G}_{RO}$ (G_{RO}) and the frequency that is detected enable the corresponding position of the proton to be determined (Figure 4-2).

Two user-selectable parameters determine the spatial resolution in the readout direction: the field of view (*FOV*) in the readout direction and the number of readout data points in the matrix. The number of readout data points together with the total sampling time determines the Nyquist frequency for the measurement (equation [2-2]). G_{RO} is defined so that protons located at the edge of the *FOV* precess at the Nyquist frequency (Figure 4-3). Smaller *FOV* are achieved by increasing G_{RO}, keeping the Nyquist frequency and thus the total receiver bandwidth constant:

$$\Delta\omega_{RO} = 2 * \omega_{NQ} = \gamma\Delta(G_{RO} * FOV) \qquad [4-3]$$

It is possible to reduce the Nyquist frequency for the measurement by reducing the total sampling time used to measure the signal. This reduces the frequency content per pixel in the final image and the background noise contributing to the measurement. In order to maintain the correct spatial resolution within the image, the readout gradient is reduced, in accordance with equation [4-3]. Regardless of the frequency resolution, the final spatial resolution is measured in mm/pixel:

$$\text{Pixel size in readout direction} = FOV/\text{Readout Matrix} \qquad [4-4]$$

In other words, while the Hz/pixel frequency content in the image is determined directly by the Nyquist frequency, the mm/pixel spatial resolution is affected only by the *FOV*.

4.3 PHASE ENCODING

The third direction in an MR image is the phase encoding direction. It is visualized along with the readout direction in an image (see Figure 4-3). The phase encoding gradient, $\mathbf{G}_{PE}$, is perpendicular to both $\mathbf{G}_{SS}$ and $\mathbf{G}_{RO}$ and is the only gradient that changes amplitude during the data

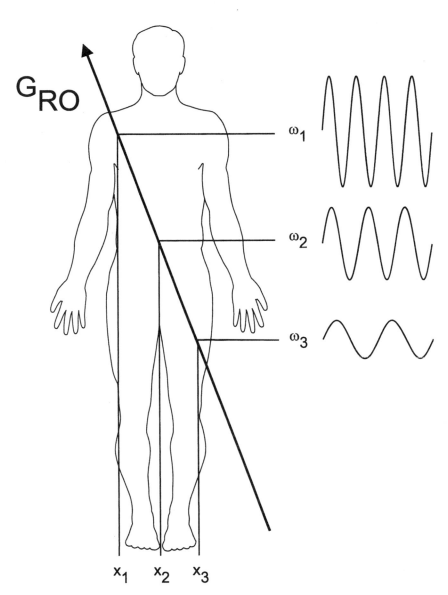

Figure 4-2. Readout process. Following excitation, each proton within the excited volume precesses at the same frequency. During detection of the echo, a gradient (G_{RO}) is applied causing a variation in the frequencies for the protons generating the echo signal. The frequency of precession ω_i for each proton depends upon its position x_i according to equation [4-1]. Frequencies measured from the echo are mapped to the corresponding position.

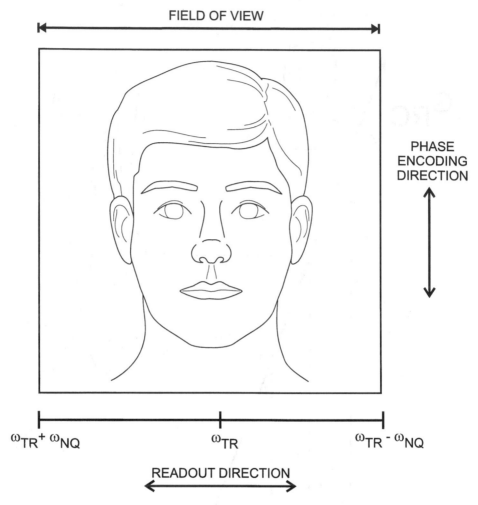

FIELD OF VIEW

PHASE ENCODING DIRECTION

$\omega_{TR} + \omega_{NQ}$ ω_{TR} $\omega_{TR} - \omega_{NQ}$

READOUT DIRECTION

Figure 4-3. Readout process. In any image, one of the visualized directions is the readout direction and the other is phase encoding direction. A proton located at the edge of the FOV in the readout direction precesses at the Nyquist frequency above or below the transmitter frequency. Changing the *FOV* of the image changes the spatial resolution (mm per pixel) but not the frequency resolution (Hz per pixel).

acquisition loop of a standard two-dimensional (2D) imaging sequence. Any signal amplitude variation detected from one acquisition to the next is assumed to be caused by the action of G_{PE} during the measurement.

The principle of phase encoding is based on the fact that the proton precession is periodic in nature. Prior to application of G_{PE}, a proton within a slice precesses at the base frequency ω_0. In the presence of G_{PE}, its precessional frequency increases or decreases according to equation [4-1]. Once G_{PE} is turned off, the proton returns to its original frequency, but is ahead or behind in phase relative to its previous state. The amount of induced phase shift depends on the magnitude and duration of G_{PE} that the proton experienced. Protons located at different positions in the phase encoding direction experience different amounts of phase shift for the same G_{PE} pulse (Figure 4-4). A proton located at the edge of the chosen *FOV* experiences the maximum amount of phase shift from each phase encoding step. The MR image information is obtained by repeating the slice excitation and signal detection multiple times, each with a different amplitude of G_{PE}. The second Fourier transformation in the image converts signal amplitude at each readout frequency from a function of G_{PE} to a function of phase.

The spatial resolution in the phase encoding direction depends on two user-selectable parameters, the *FOV* in the phase encoding direction and the number of phase encoding steps in the matrix, N_{PE}. The *FOV* is determined by the change in G_{PE} from one step to the next. For a proton located at the chosen *FOV*, each phase encoding step induces one-half cycle (180°) of phase change relative to the previous phase encoding step, assuming a constant pulse duration (Figure 4-5). N_{PE} determines the total number of cycles of phase change ($N_{PE}/2$) produced at the edge of the *FOV* and thus the maximum frequency (ω_{NQ}) in the phase encoding direction for the given pulse duration. The spatial resolution in the phase encoding direction is measured in mm/pixel:

$$\text{Pixel size in phase encoding direction} = FOV/N_{PE} \qquad [4\text{-}5]$$

Increased resolution is obtained by reducing the *FOV* or by increasing N_{PE}. The *FOV* reduction is accomplished by increasing the gradient amplitude change from one G_{PE} to the next. The *FOV* in the phase encoding direction is not required to be the same as the *FOV* in the readout direction.

4.4   DATA ACQUISITION TECHNIQUES

The previous sections described the process of spatial localization of the MR signal to a slice. For most MR applications, information from many slices is measured in order to image large volumes of tissue. Several approaches are used for data acquisition that balance the desire for good spatial resolution with maintaining reasonable scan times.

The most common measurement technique is 2D-multislice imaging. One line of data is acquired for each slice prior to measurement of a

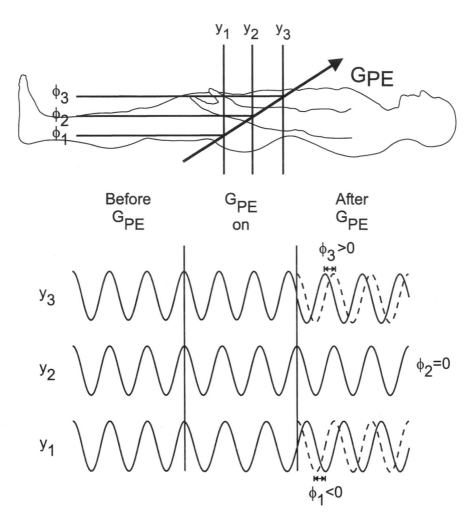

Figure 4-4. Concept of phase encoding. Prior to application of G_{PE}, all protons precess at the same frequency. When G_{PE} is applied, a proton increases or decreases its precessional frequency, depending on its position y_i. A proton located at $y_i = 0$ (y_2) experiences no effect from G_{PE} and no change in frequency or phase ($\phi_2 = 0$). A proton located at y_3 precesses faster while G_{PE} is applied. Once G_{PE} is turned off, the proton precesses at its original frequency, but is ahead of the reference frequency (dashed curve); that is, a phase shift ϕ_3 has been induced to the proton by G_{PE}. A proton located at y_1 decreases its frequency while G_{PE} is applied. Once G_{PE} is turned off, it precesses at its original frequency but is behind the reference by a phase shift of ϕ_1.

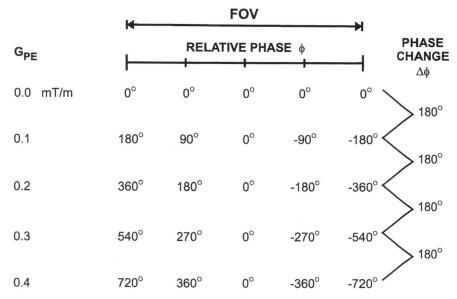

Figure 4-5. Phase encoding process. A proton at the edge of the *FOV* in the phase encoding direction undergoes 180° of phase change Δϕ from one phase encoding step to the next. Each point within the *FOV* undergoes progressively less phase change for the same gradient amplitude. A proton at isocenter never experiences any phase change. The change in gradient amplitude (0.1 mT/m) from one phase encoding step to the next depends on the particular *FOV* chosen.

second line of data from any slice. The *TR* specified by the user is the time between successive excitation pulses for a given slice. The slice loop or minimum *TR* per slice is the actual time required for the hardware to perform all the steps necessary to acquire a line of raw data. In general, the slice loop is much shorter than *TR*, allowing excitation and detection of many slices to be performed within one *TR* time period. Typically, one line of data is acquired from each slice during each *TR* time period (Figure 4-6a). The total number of lines of data collected for each slice depends on the number of phase encoding steps and the number of acquisitions N_{AQ} desired for signal averaging. The total scan time is *TR* times the total number of lines:

$$\text{Scan time}_{\text{multislice}} = TR * N_{AQ} * N_{PE} \qquad [4\text{-}6]$$

At the midpoint of a scan using a multislice collection scheme, each image has N_{PE} lines of raw data, each with the requested number of acquisitions. Note that the number of slices does not affect the total scan time; however, the maximum number of slices is limited by *TR*. The

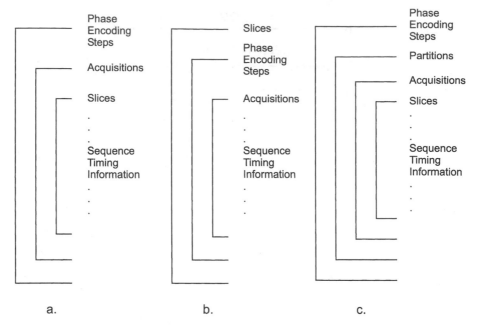

Figure 4-6. Slice loop structures. Three slice loop structures are commonly used in imaging techniques: (*a*) 2D multislice loop. The slice loop is the innermost loop. Each slice is excited and signal detected prior to any slice being excited a second time for purposes of signal averaging or phase encoding. This loop structure is the most common. (*b*) 2D sequential loop. The slice loop is the outermost loop. All information for a given slice is acquired prior to any excitation for a different slice. (*c*) 3D loop. This is a 2D multislice loop with an additional loop, the partitions loop, included within the phase encoding loop. Each signal is detected following application of both the phase encoding and partition gradient pulses.

multislice technique provides the most efficient data collection process for a given *TR*.

Another 2D data acquisition technique commonly used in MRI is the sequential slice technique. In this technique, all information for a slice is acquired before acquiring any information for another slice (Figure 4-6*b*). Only one line of data is measured during each *TR* time period. For this technique, the number of slices, N_{SLICE}, directly affects the scan time. The total scan time is thus:

$$\text{Scan time}_{\text{sequential slice}} = TR * N_{\text{AQ}} * N_{\text{PE}} * N_{\text{SLICE}} \qquad [4\text{-}7]$$

At the midpoint of a scan using the sequential slice method, all the data for one-half the requested number of slices has been acquired.

A third data acquisition technique is 3D-volume acquisition, which is, in essence, a double phase encoding technique. For 3D-volume imaging, tissue volumes of 30–150 mm are excited as compared to 3–10 mm in 2D imaging. In addition, a second phase encoding table is applied in the slice selection direction to partition or subdivide the volume into individual slices (Figure 4-6c). Each echo is acquired following application of encoding gradients in both the phase encoding and slice selection directions. For each excitation volume, the number of slices is determined by the number of partitions N_{PART}. The total scan time is:

$$\text{Scan time}_{3D} = TR * N_{AQ} * N_{PE} * N_{PART} \qquad [4\text{-}8]$$

The advantages of volume acquisition techniques are that the slices within a volume are contiguous and that the detected signal is based on the total volume excited rather than the effective slice thickness. Because of the potentially long scan times, 3D volume acquisition techniques are usually gradient echo or turbo spin echo sequences and are limited to one or two volumes.

One data collection scheme, known as the *half acquisition* or *half Fourier technique*, takes advantage of the intrinsic symmetry of the raw data to reduce the scan time. Because the negative and positive amplitude G_{PE} induce opposite polarity phase shifts to the protons (see Figure 4-4), the raw data matrix has a symmetry known as *Hermitian symmetry*. In the half Fourier approach, only 60% (all of the negative amplitude and the lowest positive amplitude G_{PE}) of the raw data matrix is measured. The maximum amplitude G_{PE} and the change in G_{PE} between each acquisition are the same as for a standard acquisition, which maintains the spatial resolution and FOV, respectively. The positive G_{PE} data are used for phase correction as well as contrast in the image. The missing raw data (high positive amplitude G_{PE}) are extrapolated from the measured data through the Hermitian symmetry prior to Fourier transformation. The resulting image has the same FOV and resolution as that from a full raw data matrix, but the scan time is 40% less. The problems with the half Fourier technique are a loss in S/N due to the reduced number of detected lines and an enhanced sensitivity to artifacts due to the replication of the information.

4.5   RAW DATA AND IMAGE DATA MATRICES

Two types of matrices are used in MRI: raw data and image data. The *raw data matrix* consists of the digitized data measured for a given echo from a given slice. The MR signal is detected using a quadrature detector consisting of two orthogonal channels. The digitized signals are stored as a complex data array with the real and imaginary parts corresponding to each detector channel. Each detected signal for a given echo corresponds to a row and each row differs by the value of G_{PE} applied prior to detection. The rows are typically displayed in order of increasing phase encoding amplitude from top to bottom. The raw data matrix is thus a grid of points with the readout direction displayed in the horizontal direction and the phase encoding direction displayed in the vertical direction. Its dimensions depend on the number of readout data points and the number of phase encoding steps (Figure 4-7a).

All the information necessary to reconstruct an image is contained within the raw data matrix. While each data point contributes to all aspects (frequency, phase, and amplitude) of every location within the slice, some data points emphasize different features in the final image. The maximum signal content is located in the central portion of the raw data matrix. These lines are acquired with low amplitude G_{PE} and provide the contrast in the image. The outer portions of the raw data matrix have relatively low signal amplitude and are acquired with either high positive amplitude or high negative amplitude G_{PE}. These gradients produce high frequencies and provide edge definition to the resultant image (Figure 4-8).

An alternate way to describe the raw data matrix is called the *k space formalism*. The array of raw data points is treated as a grid of points (k_x, k_y) where each k_x value corresponds to a different complex data point in the readout direction and each k_y value corresponds to a different phase encoding gradient amplitude. Each (k_x, k_y) data point undergoes a different and unique amount of total phase change in both the readout and phase encoding directions. The point $k_x = k_y = 0$, referred to as the origin of k space, is the maximum data point for the raw data matrix ($G_{PE} = 0$, maximum data point of the echo). Using k space terminology, contrast in the image is primarily determined by data in the center while edge definition is primarily determined by data at the edges of k space. The k space formalism provides a convenient way to describe ordering methods to acquire raw data.

Figure 4-7. (*a*) Raw data matrix, real portion. The raw data matrix has dimensions of N_{PE} * number of readout data points. Each row is a measured signal at a particular G_{PE}. The number of rows corresponds to N_{PE}. Signals acquired with high negative amplitude G_{PE} are displayed at the top, low amplitude G_{PE} in the middle, and high positive

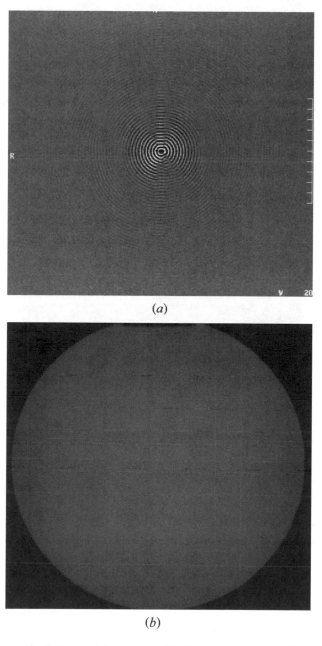

(a)

(b)

amplitude G_{PE} at the bottom of the matrix. Each column corresponds to a data point sampled at a different time following the excitation pulse. (b) Image data matrix, magnitude. The image data is obtained by performing a 2D Fourier transformation on the data set displayed in Figure 4-7a. The rows and columns correspond to the phase encoding and readout directions. The specification of rows and columns as readout and

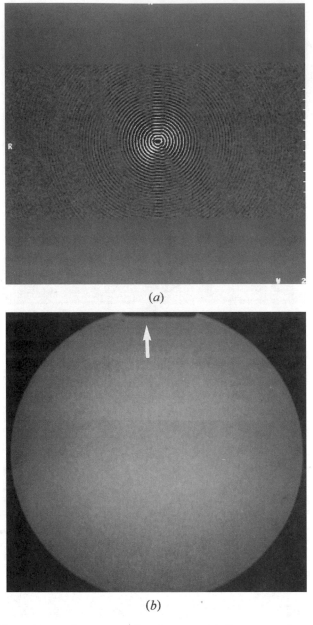

(a)

(b)

Figure 4-8. Raw data and corresponding images. (a) Same raw data set as Figure 4-7a except that 50% of the phase encoding steps are missing, the most positive 64 and the most negative 64 steps. (b) Image data of Figure 4-8a. The image intensity is approximately the same as Figure 4-7b, but there is a small loss of edge definition, exhibited as blurring at the edge of the phantom (arrow). (c) Same raw data set as Figure 4-7a except the central 32 phase encoding steps, corresponding to 12.5% of the total. (d) Image data of Figure 4-8c. The image intensity (central portion of the phantom) is virtually absent, while the edges of the phantom are present.

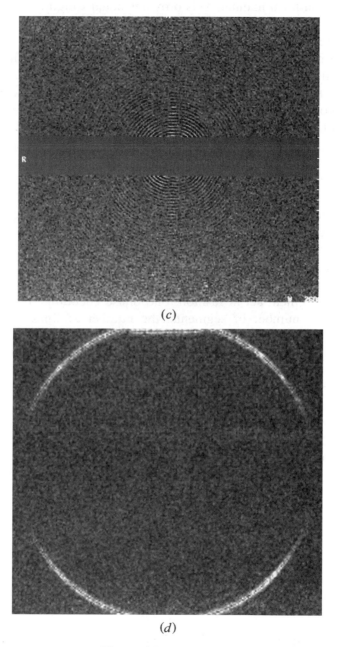

(c)

(d)

Figure 4-8. (*Continued*)

In general, it is desirable to acquire the raw data (sample k space) in a relatively uniform manner. This provides equal weight to both contrast and edge definition in the final image. However, the order in which the lines of the raw data matrix are acquired is somewhat arbitrary. The traditional method for data collection is sequential filling. The raw data matrix is filled, one line at a time, with adjacent k_y lines acquired sequentially in time beginning with the most negative G_{PE} and ending with the most positive G_{PE}. The step $G_{PE} = 0$ occurs halfway through the data collection (Figure 4-9a). Other methods are used when additional contrast control is required or for special applications. Reordered k space refers to methods of data collection where the raw data are acquired in a nonsequential fashion. Centric ordering acquires the low amplitude phase encoding steps earliest in the scan, with higher amplitude phase encoding steps acquired later (Figure 4-9b). Variations on sequential and centric ordering are possible, in which the center of k space is acquired at other times of the scan. Another useful approach for data collection is the segmented method, in which successive echoes in the scan measure lines from different regions or segments of k space. Data are collected in a segment serial fashion, one phase encoding step from each segment. The number of segments, the number of lines per segment, and the order of acquisition may be independently varied (Figure 4-9c).

The image data or display matrix is obtained via the 2D Fourier transform from the raw data matrix. The image matrix is a frequency and phase map of the proton signal intensity from a volume element weighted by the T1 and T2 values of the tissues contained within the volume. The frequencies and phases are determined by the location of the volume element. While the Fourier transformation contains information regarding both the magnitude and phase of the measured signals, the normal image matrix contains only magnitude information. Although they must be the same dimension as the raw data matrix, image matrices are usually displayed as square images with readout as one direction and phase encoding as the other direction in the image (Figure 4-7b). The choice of rows and columns for readout and phase encoding is at the operator's discretion and is made to minimize artifacts in the area of interest. The maximum dimensions in the image matrix normally correspond to the chosen FOV in each direction.

4.6   FREQUENCY SELECTIVE EXCITATION

Chapter 2 presented the concepts of rf excitation and resonance absorption by the protons. In MR, the rf energy is applied as pulsed excitation,

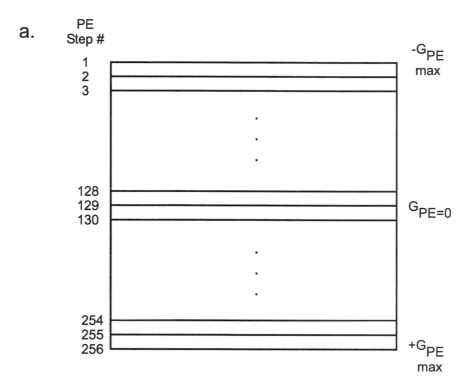

Figure 4-9. Raw data collection schemes. Each line of k space (phase encoding step) corresponds to a measured MR signal. Three methods of raw data collection are shown: (*a*) Sequential data collection. Lines of k space are acquired serially in time with the data from the maximum negative G_{PE} acquired first and the data from the maximum positive G_{PE} acquired last. The center of k space (G_{PE} = 0 mT/m step) is acquired halfway through the data collection period. This is the traditional data collection method. (*b*) Centric ordering. Lines of k space are acquired serially beginning at the center of k space then in increasing G_{PE} amplitudes with alternating polarity. (*c*) Segmented data collection. Lines of k space are acquired in groups or segments. The example here shows three segments. One line of data is acquired from each segment before a second line is acquired from any segment. The center of k space is acquired at a time dependent on the number of lines per segment, number of segments, and the order of acquisition within a segment and between segments. *Illustration continued on following page.*

with a center frequency, duration, shape, amplitude, and phase defined for each pulse. Pulses may be applied using amplitude modulation, where the energy is distributed to all frequencies at the same time during the pulse, or using frequency modulation, where frequencies are sequentially excited during application of the pulse. The center frequency of the pulse is normally chosen as the resonant frequency for the particular collection of protons under observation. The duration and shape

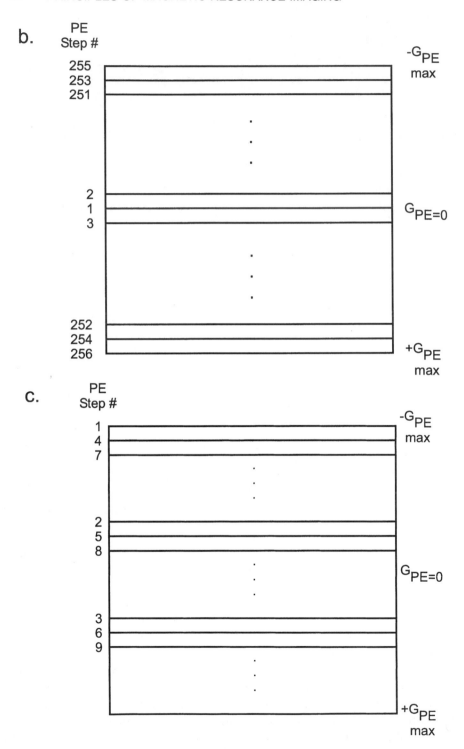

Figure 4-9. (*Continued*)

of the pulse determine the bandwidth or range of frequencies on either side of the center frequency that are excited by the pulse. The phase of the pulse defines the effective orientation of the rf energy (see Figure 2-2) and determines the axis of rotation for the net magnetization under the influence of the pulse. The pulse amplitude, or more precisely, the amplitude integral, determines the amount of rotation that the protons undergo (flip angle). In addition, the pulse amplitude determines the amount of energy that the protons absorb. For most MRI applications, uniform excitation of the frequencies encompassed by the pulse is normally the preferred result; that is, the pulse excites all frequencies equally within its selected range.

A common means of classification of rf pulses is by the pulse shape, referred to as the *pulse envelope*, that is broadcast and the resulting bandwidth of frequencies that are excited by the pulse. The rf envelope consists of a time-varying set of complex data points, typically several hundred in number. These digital points are converted to an analog signal prior to mixing with the carrier frequency and broadcasting. *Nonselective* pulses, also known as *rectangular* or *hard pulses*, are of short duration and constant amplitude and excite a broad frequency range with a uniform amplitude. They are usually used to determine the resonant frequency of the patient. Nonselective pulses may also be used in a series of pulses applied in a very short time period, known as a *composite pulse* (see Chapter 7). Strictly speaking, "nonselective" pulses are frequency selective since the pulsed nature of the excitation limits the frequency bandwidth that can be incorporated into the pulse.

The other class of rf envelopes are *frequency selective* or *soft pulses*. Frequency selective pulses do not have constant amplitude at all times or at all frequencies during broadcast. The transmitter duration is longer than for a nonselective pulse, allowing for a narrower frequency bandwidth. In MRI, most rf pulses used are frequency selective pulses because it is desirable to focus the excitation on narrow regions of tissue for most applications. The frequency bandwidth of the pulse determines the slice thickness, according to equation [4-2], and the slice profile.

For standard slice selective excitation pulses, uniform amplitude and phase excitation throughout the slice is necessary. This is easiest accomplished using an amplitude-modulated pulse of short duration. For a pulse to excite a particular frequency, that frequency must be included within its bandwidth. As more frequencies at the same phase are included in a pulse, the amplitude variations as a function of time (the pulse shape) approach a function known as a sinc function, an infinite function that contains all possible frequencies (Figure 4-10). Due to the

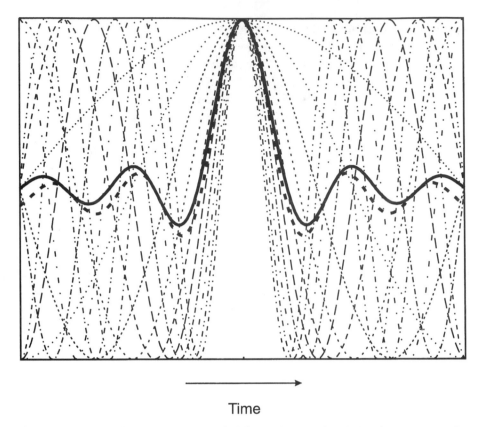

Time

Figure 4-10. A series of sine waves of different frequencies all in phase at one point in time sum to give an approximation (broken dark line) to an infinite sinc function (solid dark line).

short duration of the pulse and its limited bandwidth (the pulse bandwidth is inversely related to its duration), the actual pulse shape used for slice selective pulses is a truncated sinc function. This truncation causes the frequency cutoff to be less than ideal and has two important consequences: frequencies outside the desired bandwidth are excited as well as those within the bandwidth, and the dropoff of the excitation, known as the *pulse profile*, is not rectangular but has sloped sides. The extraneous excitation can be minimized by filtering the sinc function or mathematically forcing it to zero at the edges. This reduces the total power contained within the pulse, but accentuates the sloped nature of the pulse profile.

The response of the protons to pulsed excitation is complicated and requires the use of linear response theory for a complete description, which is beyond the scope of this book. However, in general, amplitude-modulated rf excitation pulses are subject to two competing criteria:

1. Short duration pulses require high peak pulse amplitudes to achieve the same pulse area (flip angle). Depending on the particular rf amplifier and transmitter coil, the maximum power that can be broadcast is limited.

2. Sinc functions produce rectangular, phase coherent excitation profiles only with low flip angles (<30°). High amplitude pulses such as 90° or 180° pulses have excitation profiles that are significantly nonrectangular. Manufacturers strive to provide uniform excitation profiles, subject to criteria 1. Specific questions about particular rf pulse profiles should be addressed to the individual manufacturer.

Two additional rf profiles are used for specific applications. Gaussian pulses are often used for frequency-selective saturation pulses such as fat suppression or magnetization transfer suppression due to a narrower excitation bandwidth (see Chapter 7). These pulses have excitation pro-

a.   b.

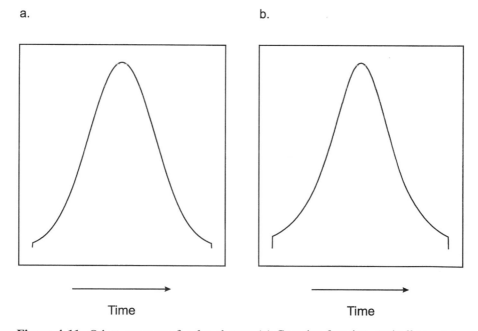

Time   Time

Figure 4-11. Other common rf pulse shapes. (*a*) Gaussian function, typically used for frequency-selective saturation pulses (fat saturation, magnetization transfer suppression). (*b*) Hyperbolic secant, often used for inversion pulses.

files that follow a Gaussian shape, which is narrower than the sinc function. Another pulse shape is known as *hyperbolic secant*. This pulse is usually applied as a frequency- or phase-modulated adiabatic pulse and produces very good 180° inversion pulses at low transmitter amplitude levels. Hyperbolic secant pulses are often used in inversion recovery sequences (see Chapter 5), but they have phase variations that make them unsuitable for use as a refocusing pulse. Figure 4-11 illustrates these pulse shapes.

Pulse Sequences

A pulse sequence is the measurement technique by which an MR image is obtained. It contains the hardware instructions necessary to acquire the data in the desired manner. The signal intensity produced from a volume element of tissue is determined by both the measurement parameters directly selected by the user and the variables dictated by the pulse sequence. The effect of the measurement parameters is discussed in more detail in Chapter 6. Some parameters of a pulse sequence (e.g., minimum *TR*, *FOV*) depend on how the manufacturer has implemented the technique (e.g., gradient pulse duration) while others (e.g., maximum gradient amplitude, gradient rise time) are determined by limitations of the hardware.

One of the more confusing aspects of MRI is the variety of pulse sequences available from the different equipment manufacturers. In addition, similar sequences may be known by a variety of names by the same manufacturer. As a result, comparison of techniques and protocols between manufacturers is often difficult due to differences in sequence implementation. An accurate description and comparison of techniques between manufacturers would require knowledge of proprietary information. This chapter describes several pulse sequences commonly used in imaging by all manufacturers and some of the general characteristics of each one. In addition, where appropriate, the common acronyms used by some of the major manufacturers for the sequences are included.

Comparison of pulse sequences is facilitated by the use of timing diagrams. Timing diagrams are schematic representations of the basic steps performed by the different hardware components during sequence execution. Although there may be stylistic differences in the diagrams prepared by different authors, the general features are the same for all diagrams (Figure 5-1). Elapsed time during sequence execution is indicated left to right along the horizontal axis. The vertical separation between lines is employed only for visualization. Each line corresponds to a different hardware component. At a minimum, four lines are used to describe any pulse sequence: one representing the radiofrequency (rf)

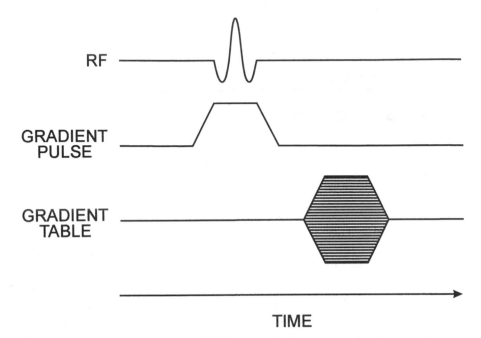

RF

GRADIENT
PULSE

GRADIENT
TABLE

TIME

Figure 5-1. Simple timing diagram. The horizontal axis is time during sequence execution. Each line corresponds to a different hardware component (rf transmitter, gradient amplifier, or ADC sampling period). Activity for a component is shown as a deviation from the baseline. Times during sequence execution when more than one hardware component is active (e.g., rf transmitter and gradient) are illustrated as activity in both lines. Gradient activity that does not change from measurement to measurement (e.g., slice selection amplitude) is shown as a constant deviation from baseline. Gradient activity that changes from measurement to measurement (e.g., phase encoding amplitude) is shown as a hashed region to illustrate multiple values.

transmitter and one representing each gradient (labeled as G_X, G_Y, G_Z, or G_{SLICE}, G_{READ}, and G_{PHASE}). Additional lines may be added to indicate other activity such as analog-to-digital converter (ADC) sampling. Activity for a particular component such as a gradient pulse is shown as a deviation above or below the horizontal line. Simultaneous activity from more than one component such as the rf transmitter and slice selection gradient is indicated by nonzero activity from both lines at the same horizontal position. Constant amplitude gradient pulses are shown as simple deviations from zero. Gradient tables such as for phase encoding are represented as hashed regions. Timing diagrams typically represent the hardware activity for one slice loop of the pulse sequence. Specific details regarding exact timings, individual gradient amplitudes, or looping structures are not included as much of this information is determined by the specific measurement parameters or is proprietary to the various manufacturers. The generic nature of the representations makes timing diagrams suitable to represent classes of pulse sequences when making comparisons between the various measurement techniques.

5.1   SPIN ECHO SEQUENCES

A commonly used pulse sequence in MR imaging is a spin echo sequence. It has at least two rf pulses, an excitation pulse (often called the *alpha* (α) *pulse*) and one or more 180° refocusing pulses that generate the spin echo(es). A refocusing pulse is required for evey echo produced. Spin echo sequences also utilize gradient pulses of opposite polarity in the readout and slice selection directions to refocus the protons at the same time as the spin echo. Spoiler gradients are used following signal detection to dephase any residual transverse magnetization and minimize spurious echoes. In a spin echo sequence, the repetition time, *TR*, is the time between successive excitation pulses for a given slice. The echo time, *TE*, is the time from the excitation pulse to the echo maximum. A multislice loop structure is used to acquire signals from multiple slices within one *TR* time period. Table 5-1 lists some of the common names for spin echo sequences.

Three types of spin echo sequences are commonly used: standard single echo, standard multiecho, and echo train spin echo. Standard single echo sequences are generally used to produce T1-weighted images when acquired with relatively short *TR* and *TE* (less than 700 ms and 30 ms, respectively). A multislice loop structure is used with a single pair of excitation and refocusing pulses applied per slice loop. A single phase encoding amplitude is applied per excitation pulse. Each echo within the scan is measured at the selected *TE* but with a different amplitude for G_{PE} (Figure 5-2). Any raw data signal intensity variations from measurement to measurement are due to changes in G_{PE} only. Following reconstruction, amplitude variations between tissues in the image are the result of differences between tissue specific properties (proton density, T1, T2).

Standard multiecho sequences apply extra 180° refocusing rf pulses following a single excitation pulse. Each refocusing pulse produces a spin echo, each one at a different *TE* defined by the user. A single G_{PE} is used per rf excitation pulse (Figure 5-3). Differences in raw data signal intensity at each *TE* are still due to differences in G_{PE} only. Raw data signal intensity changes from echo to echo (*TE* to *TE*) are due to T2

Table 5-1 Spin Echo Pulse Sequence Acronyms

	Single Echo	Multiple Echo	Echo Train Spin Echo
Siemens	Single spin echo	Spin echo, Double echo	Turbo spin echo (TSE), Half Fourier acquisition turbo spin echo (HASTE)
GE	Spin echo	Multiecho multiplanar (MEMP), Variable echo multiplanar (VEMP)	Fast spin echo (FSE), Single shot FSE (SS-FSE)
Philips	Spin echo, modified spin echo	Multiple spin echo (MSE)	Turbo spin echo (TSE), Ultrafast spin echo (UFSE)
Picker	Spin echo, throughput heightened rapid increased flip T2 (THRIFT), Phase symmeterized rapid increased flip spin echo (PRISE)	Multiecho, throughput heightened rapid increased flip T2 (THRIFT)	Fast spin echo (FSE)

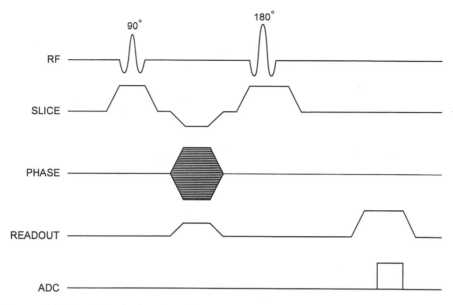

Figure 5-2. Standard single echo spin echo sequence timing diagram. These sequences are characterized by a single 180° refocusing pulse, a single detected echo, and a single phase encoding table. The TE time is measured from the middle of the excitation pulse to the center of the echo.

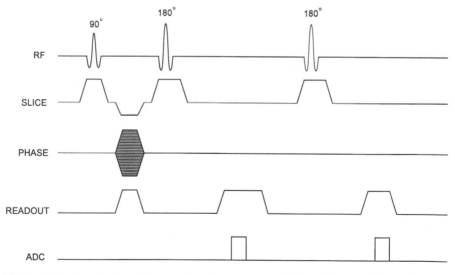

Figure 5-3. Standard multiecho spin echo sequence timing diagram. Two echoes are illustrated. Additional echoes may be generated by adding additional 180° rf pulses, slice selection gradient pulses, readout gradient pulses, and ADC sampling times. Note the single phase encoding gradient table. Both *TE* times are measured from the middle of the excitation pulse to the center of the respective echo.

relaxation. Multiecho sequences are used to produce proton density-weighted images at short *TE* (less than 30 ms) and T2-weighted images at long *TE* (greater than 80 ms) when *TR* is long enough to allow relatively complete T1 relaxation for most tissues (2000 ms or longer).

The third type of spin echo sequence is known as echo train spin echo (ETSE). It is based on the RARE (rapid acquisition with relaxation enhancement) technique for imaging. The ETSE sequences are similar to standard multiecho sequences in that multiple 180° pulses are applied to produce multiple echoes following a single excitation pulse. However, each echo signal is acquired with a different G_{PE} as well as a different *TE* (Figure 5-4). The image is produced using some or all of the measured echoes as determined by the sequence design. The echo train length corresponds to the number of echoes used. A segmented gradient table is used with one echo from each segment acquired as part of the echo train for each rf pulse. The advantage of the ETSE technique is

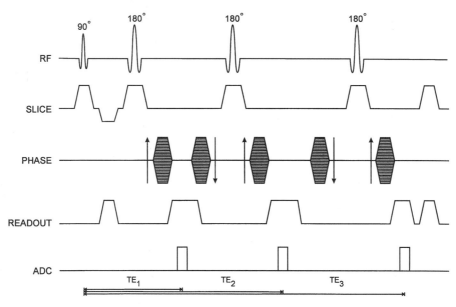

Figure 5-4. Echo train spin echo sequence timing diagram. A three-segment (echo train length of 3) version is illustrated, each with $N_{PE}/3$ values of G_{PE} per segment to acquire N_{PE} total lines of raw data. The arrows beside the G_{PE} tables indicate the direction in which the phase encoding values change from one excitation pulse to the next. Gradient tables on opposite sides of the ADC sampling time have equal amplitudes but opposite polarity. The effective *TE* is the *TE* (1, 2, or 3) during which the $G_{PE} = 0$ lines of data are acquired.

that the data collection process is more efficient and the scan time is shorter:

$$\text{Scan time}_{\text{EchoTrainSpinEcho}} = TR * N_{\text{AQ}} * N_{\text{PE}}/\text{Echo train length} \quad [5\text{-}1]$$

The contrast in ETSE sequences is determined primarily by the echoes detected at or near $G_{\text{PE}} = 0$ and the *TE*s for these echoes. The contrast is considered to be based on an effective *TE* since there are echoes with different *TE*s contributing to the final image. This use of multiple *TE*s in the creation of the image makes ETSE sequences unsuitable for use when subtle differences in *TE* between tissues are responsible for the image contrast.

While ETSE sequences can be used to produce T1-weighted images, their most common application has been to produce T2-weighted images. This is due to the significant reduction in scan time that can be achieved for long *TR* scans when modest echo train lengths are used. While echo train lengths less than 10 are typically used for brain and spine imaging, very long echo trains (100 or more) can be used in abdominal imaging to acquire T2-weighted images in less than one second. Termed *snapshot* or *ultrafast ETSE*, the scan times are sufficiently short to freeze bowel motion, yet provide excellent T2 contrast between tissues.

5.2 INVERSION RECOVERY SEQUENCES

The inversion recovery (IR) sequence is a variation of the spin echo sequence. It is a spin echo sequence with an additional 180° pulse, usually slice selective, applied prior to the initial excitation pulse. The 180° pulse inverts **M** for the protons within the slice, producing enhanced T1 sensitivity at the time of the excitation pulse. The inversion time, *TI*, is a user-selectable delay time between the 180° pulse and the excitation pulse and determines the amount of T1 relaxation that occurs between the two pulses. A standard phase encoding gradient table is used, and *TE* is defined as for spin echo sequences (Figure 5-5). Table 5-2 lists common names and features for inversion recovery sequences. Inversion recovery sequences require long *TR* times to allow maximal T1 relaxation between successive excitation rf pulses. Insufficient *TR* causes loss of signal due to saturation for tissues with long T1 relaxation times such as fluids.

Three sequence variations are used for IR sequences. The echo train inversion recovery sequence combines features of the normal IR and the

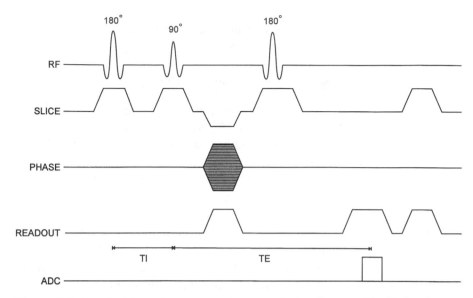

Figure 5-5. Standard inversion recovery sequence timing diagram. The *TI* time is measured from the middle of the inversion pulse to the excitation pulse. The *TE* is measured from the middle of the excitation pulse to the center of the echo.

ETSE sequences. The 180° inversion pulse is applied prior to a ETSE acquisition sequence rather than a normal spin echo sequence. The contrast obtained in a echo train IR sequence is based on the *TI* and the tissue *TI* times as in the IR sequence, while the echo train length and effective *TE* have equivalent effects to these parameters in the ETSE sequence (Figure 5-6). The second modification is the looping mode for multislice imaging. If the *TI* time is relatively short, all rf pulses are applied to and signal is detected from a slice before progressing to another slice. If the *TI* time is relatively long, all inversion rf pulses are applied in order, then the excitation and refocusing pulses are applied. This allows for more efficient data collection during one *TR* time period.

The third type of sequence modification is determined by the image reconstruction process. The inversion of **M** by the 180° rf pulse allows for the generation of negative amplitude signals. Short *TI* times allow minimal T1 relaxation between the inversion and excitation rf pulses. Most tissues will have **M** inverted at the time of the excitation pulse. Long *TI* times allow more complete relaxation of tissues between the two pulses, producing positive values for **M**. Intermediate *TI* gives a mixture of positive and negative **M**, depending on the specific tissue T1 values and *TI* (Figure 5-7). During image reconstruction, the phase of **M** can be incorporated into the pixel intensity. Termed *phase sensitive*

Table 5-2 Inversion Recovery Pulse Sequence Acronyms

	Standard Inversion Recovery	Echo Train Inversion Recovery	Interleaved Excitation	Magnitude Reconstruction	Phase Sensitive Reconstruction
Siemens	IR	TurboIR	Interleaved	Absolute value, magnitude (standard)	TrueIR
GE	Multiplanar IR (MPIR)	Fast multiplanar IR (FMPIR)	Nonsequential		—
Philips	IR	IR-turbo spin echo (IR–TSE)	—	Modulus (standard)	Real
Picker	IR	IR	Slice Interleaved		—

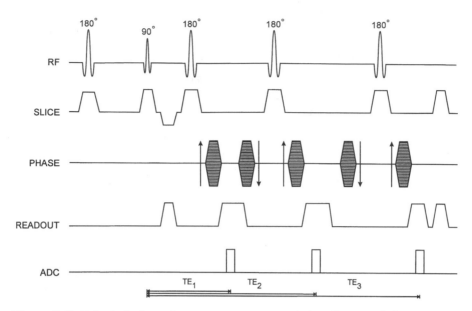

Figure 5-6. Echo train inversion recovery sequence timing diagram. A three-segment (echo train length of 3) version is illustrated, each segment with $N_{PE}/3$ values for G_{PE}. The *TI* time is measured from the middle of the inversion pulse to the excitation pulse. The effective *TE* is the *TE* (1, 2, or 3) during which the $G_{PE} = 0$ lines of data are acquired.

IR, these images have negative pixel values for tissues with inverted **M**. These are produced by tissues with long T1 values at short *TI* times. Background air is assigned a midrange pixel value. Alternately, the phase of **M** can be ignored in the final image. Termed *absolute value* or *magnitude IR*, these images have pixel values based only on the signal magnitude. Tissues with very short or very long T1 relaxation times have high pixel values, and background air has a low pixel value.

The inversion pulse also allows for the suppression of signal through the proper choice of *TI*. If the *TI* time is chosen when the tissue of interest has no longitudinal component, then that tissue contributes no signal to the final image. This time, known as the *null time* for the tissue, is determined by the T1 relaxation time for the tissue:

$$TI_{NULL} = 0.693 * T1 \qquad [5\text{-}2]$$

assuming the *TR* time is sufficiently long. The two most common applications of IR sequences are for the suppression of cerebrospinal fluid (CSF) and fat. Normal CSF has a T1 relaxation time of approximately 3000 ms at 1.5 T. A *TI* time of 2080 ms will apply the excitation pulse

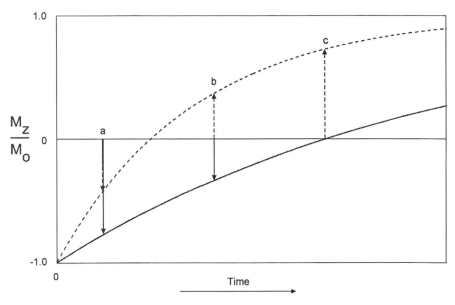

Figure 5-7. T1 recovery curves for inversion recovery sequences. The 180° inversion pulse inverts the net magnetization for all tissues. Tissue with short T1 times (dashed curve) recovers faster than tissue with long T1 (solid curve) times. For a *TI* time of (a), both tissues contribute significant negative amplitude signal. For a *TI* time of (b), the short T1 tissue contributes positive amplitude signal while the long T1 tissue contributes negative amplitude signal. For a *TI* time of (c), the short T1 tissue contributes significant positive amplitude signal and the long T1 tissue contributes no signal. If the signal polarity is considered (phase sensitive IR sequences), signal difference will be seen at all three TI times. If the signal polarity is ignored (absolute value or magnitude IR sequences), no difference in signal between the two tissues will be seen at time (b).

when the CSF magnetization has no longitudinal component and produces an image with no CSF signal. This technique, known as fluid-attentuated IR (FLAIR), allows easy visualization of gray and white matter inflammation.

Fat has a T1 relaxation time of approximately 200–250 ms at 1.5 T. If a *TI* value of 140–160 msec is selected, the excitation pulse occurs when the fat magnetization has no longitudinal component and produces an image with no fat signal. This technique is known as STIR or short TI inversion recovery. Virtually complete and uniform fat suppression throughout the imaging volume can be achieved using STIR imaging. However, it suffers from two major limitations. One is that a limited number of slices can be acquired for typical *TR*. Because of this, multiple scans are often required to obtain complete coverage of the imaging volume. The second problem occurs with the use of a T1 contrast agent.

As described in Chapter 14, a contrast agent such as Gd-DTPA shortens the T1 relaxation time for the water in tissues that absorb the agent. Tissues with long T1 values that would normally be bright in a STIR image will lose signal when the contrast agent is present as the tissue T1 approaches that of the fat tissue. Visualization of these tissues thus becomes difficult. For this reason, STIR imaging is usually not performed when contrast agents are given.

5.3   GRADIENT ECHO SEQUENCES

Gradient echo sequences are a class of imaging techniques that do not use a 180° pulse to refocus the protons. The echo signal is generated only through gradient reversal. As mentioned in Chapter 3, application of imaging gradients induce proton dephasing. Application of a second gradient pulse of the same duration and magnitude but opposite polarity reverses this dephasing and produces an echo known as a *gradient echo*. All gradient echo sequences use gradient reversal pulses in at least two directions, the slice selection and the readout directions, which generate the echo signal. Excitation angles less than 90° are normally used.

The absence of the 180° rf pulse in gradient echo sequences has several important consequences. The slice loop may be shorter than for an analogous spin echo sequence, enabling more slices to be acquired for the same *TR* if a multislice loop is used. Less total rf power is applied to the patient, so that the total rf energy deposition is lower. Additional contrast mechanisms are also possible. The static sources for proton dephasing, the $\mathbf{B}_0$ inhomogeneity and the magnetic susceptibility differences, contribute to the signal decay, so the *TE* determines the amount of T2* weighting in a gradient echo image rather than only T2 as in a spin echo image (equation [3-2]). For this reason, the overall signal level in gradient echo images will be less than for spin echo images with comparable acquisition parameters. In addition, fat and water protons within a voxel also contribute different amounts of signal, depending upon the chosen *TE*, a process known as *phase cycling* (see Chapter 8, Phase cancellation artifact). Table 5-3 lists some of the common gradient echo sequences currently in use.

The simplest gradient echo sequence is a *spoiled gradient echo* sequence. This sequence uses a spoiling scheme to dephase the transverse magnetization following signal detection. As a result, only longitudinal magnetization contributes to **M** at the time of the next rf pulse (e.g., *TR*). Spoiling may be done either by applying high amplitude gradient

Table 5-3 Gradient Echo Pulse Sequence Acronyms

	Spoiled	Refocused, Postexcitation	Refocused, Pre-excitation	Magnetization Prepared
Siemens	Fast low angle shot (FLASH)	Fast imaging with steady state precession (FISP)	Reversed FISP (PSIF)	TurboFLASH, Magnetization prepared rapid acquisition gradient echo (MP-RAGE)
GE	Spoiled GRASS (SPGR), Fast spoiled GRASS (FSPGR), Multiplanar spoiled GRASS (MPSPGR), Fast multiplanar spoiled GRASS (FMPSPGR)	Gradient acquisition in the steady state (GRASS), Fast GRASS, Multiplanar GRASS (MPGR), Fast multiplanar GRASS (FMPGR)	Steady state free precession (SSFP)	IR-prepared fast GRASS, Driven equilibrium (DE)-prepared fast GRASS
Philips	T1 contrast-enhanced FFE (T1 CE-FFE)	Fast field echo (FFE)	T2 contrast-enhanced FFE (T2 CE-FFE)	Turbo field echo (TFE)
Picker	RF-FAST	Fourier-acquired steady state (FAST)	Contrast enhanced FAST (CE-FAST)	Rapid acquisition magnetization prepared FAST (RAM-FAST)

pulses known as "spoiler" or "crusher" pulses to dephase the magnetization or by varying the phase of the rf excitation pulse in a pseudorandom fashion each application. This approach, known as *rf spoiling*, produces an incoherent addition of any residual transverse magnetization so that the only remaining coherence at the time of the next excitation pulse is in the longitudinal direction (Figure 5-8).

In many respects, the spoiled gradient echo technique is the gradient echo counterpart of the spin echo technique. However, the contrast behavior of spoiled gradient echo techniques is slightly more complicated. The *TE* determines the amount of T2* rather than T2 contrast. The combination of excitation angle and *TR* determines the amount of T1 weighting in a spoiled gradient echo image. Low excitation angle pulses impart minimal rf energy and leave most of **M** in the longitudinal direction. This allows shorter *TR* to be used without producing saturation of the protons. Proton density-weighted images are produced for small excitation angles (15–20°), relatively long *TR* (500 ms), and short *TE* (10 ms). T2* weighted images can be obtained using the same excitation angle and *TR* but a long *TE* (25 ms). Substantial T1 weighting is obtained using large excitation angles (80°), short *TR* (100–150 ms), and short *TE* (less than 10 ms). Spoiled gradient echo images may be ac-

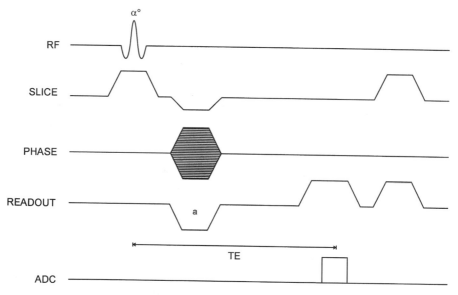

Figure 5-8. Spoiled gradient echo sequence timing diagram, 2D method. Because there is no 180° rf pulse, the polarity of the G_{RO} dephasing gradient pulse (a) is opposite that of the readout gradient pulse applied during signal detection. Gradient spoiling is illustrated at the end of the loop.

quired using any of the data acquisition techniques discussed in Chapter 4. Routine spoiled gradient echo imaging for spinal or abdominal studies uses a 2D multislice mode. A 2D sequential mode is used for MR angiography (see Chapter 10) while a 3D volume acquisition can produce very thin slices useful for multiplanar reconstruction of images in arbitrary orientations.

A second group of gradient sequences belongs to a class of techniques known as *refocused gradient echo* sequences. Refocused gradient echo sequences use a single excitation pulse with a *TR* shorter than the T2 relaxation time. Once the steady state is produced (following a few rf pulses), both longitudinal and transverse components of **M** are present at the time of the next excitation pulse. Unlike spoiled gradient echo sequences, refocused sequences apply rephasing gradient pulses in all three directions to maintain the transverse magnetization as much as possible. In addition, the excitation pulses are applied rapidly enough (short *TR*) so that spin echoes are generated that occur simultaneously with the subsequent excitation pulses. These spin echoes refocus the transverse magnetization as in spin echo imaging so that the signal amplitude in refocused pulse sequences depends strongly upon the T1 and T2 relaxation times of the tissues under observation.

Two signals can be measured from a refocused pulse scheme, one before and one after the excitation pulse (Figure 5-9). This scenario is

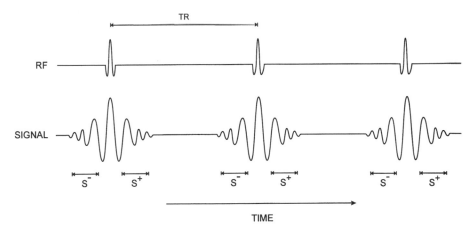

Figure 5-9. A series of equally spaced rf pulses produces spin echoes that form at the time of the subsequent rf excitation pulses. Once a steady state is reached (following several *TR* time periods), signal is induced prior to and following the excitation pulse. The pre-excitation pulse signal (S⁻) is strictly echo reformation. The postexcitation pulse signal (S⁺) is a combination of echo and free induction decay. Images can be produced from either signal or from both.

analogous to examining a normal spin echo and using the protons as they rephase prior to *TE* to produce one signal and as they dephase following *TE* to produce the other signal. In spin echo imaging, both halves of the echo are detected and are processed together. In gradient echo imaging, each half of the echo can produce an image. The two pulse sequences are complementary in their sequence timing (Figure 5-10*a,b*). The technique using the postexcitation pulse signal is conceptually similar to the spoiled gradient echo technique except for the unspoiled transverse magnetization.

Optimal contrast in refocused gradient echo sequences can only be achieved in tissues with long T1 and T2 relaxation times. Bright signals are produced by both pre- and postexcitation techniques for tissues such as cerebrospinal fluid and blood with relatively long T2 and when *TR* is short so that the transverse coherence is maintained. A difference between the two techniques is observed when using a long *TR* or for tissues with T2 that is much shorter than T1. In these cases, no transverse component to **M** is present at the time of the next excitation pulse so that the tissue contrast using a postexcitation technique is similar to that of spoiled gradient echo (based only on the longitudinal component of **M**). That is, the signal intensity for the postexcitation technique approaches that of the spoiled gradient echo at long *TR* (e.g., 500 ms). This occurs because of the equivalent loss of transverse magnetization prior to the subsequent excitation pulse, either due to natural causes or deliberate dephasing, respectively. In contrast, signal in the preexcitation technique decreases with increasing *TR* so that at long *TR*, no image is produced.

5.4 MAGNETIZATION PREPARED SEQUENCES

One difficulty in MRI is that increased spatial resolution is usually obtained at the expense of increased measurement times. Typical MRI scans require several minutes to acquire in-plane resolution of $1-2$ mm^2 pixels. By sacrificing spatial resolution, images may be obtained in $1-2$ seconds using gradient echo techniques. For example, a *TR* of 7 ms with $N_{PE} = 128$ will require 900 ms of scan time. The excitation angle must be between 5° and 10° to minimize saturation effects yet produce sufficient transverse magnetization to generate a signal. Added contrast may be obtained by manipulating the longitudinal magnetization through the application of additional rf pulses prior to the data collection period. These preparation pulses generate enhanced variations to **M** that can be

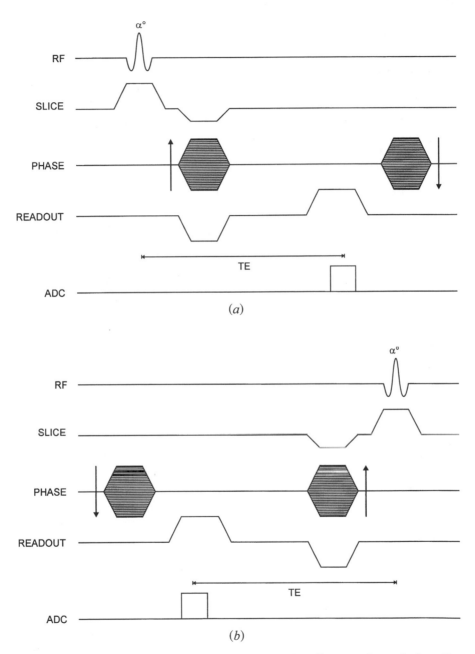

Figure 5-10. Refocused gradient echo sequence timing diagrams. Instead of spoiling the transverse magnetization, rephasing gradients are used to maintain the transverse magnetization as much as possible. (*a*) Postexcitation imaging sequence. (*b*) Pre-excitation imaging sequence.

measured during the rapid data collection time. This is the concept of magnetization prepared (MP) gradient echo sequences.

MP sequences are non-steady-state techniques in that **M** does not have the same value prior to each phase-encoding step. Each phase-encoding step is acquired at a different point in time following the preparation pulses. The resulting image contrast depends on when the $G_{PE} = 0$ step is acquired during the data collection period. The $G_{PE} = 0$ time is determined by the particular gradient table-ordering scheme used. Standard sequential ordering has the $G_{PE} = 0$ step in the middle of the phase encoding table so that the $G_{PE} = 0$ step is acquired at a time $TR * N_{Pe} * N_{AQ}/2$ into the data collection period. The contrast in this case depends on the matrix size and acquisitions. Centric ordering acquires the $G_{PE} = 0$ step at the beginning of the data collection period so that the $G_{PE} = 0$ step occurs at a time TR into the data collection period. The contrast for a centric-ordered MP sequence does not vary as dramatically with the extrinsic variables and has more predictable contrast behavior.

MP techniques can be either 2D or 3D techniques. Two-dimensional MP techniques are acquired as sequential slice techniques in that all data collection is acquired for a slice following a single set of preparation pulses. The rapid measurement times make them very insensitive to patient motion. These sequences may also be acquired using a segmented k space in order to increase spatial resolution. Three-dimensional MP techniques typically apply one preparation pulse per phase encoding entry so that the non-steady-state behavior to **M** is only present during the loop through the partitions gradient table. This enables the image contrast to be unaffected by the acquisition matrix.

Two types of preparatory schemes are used in MP sequences. For T1-weighted images, a single 180° inversion rf pulse is applied (Figure 5-11a). This pulse may be nonselective to invert all protons within the transmitter coil or slice selective to invert only the protons in the slice of interest. A delay time TI between the inversion pulse and the data collection period produces variation in longitudinal magnetization of the tissues. T1 MP sequences differ from the IR sequences described previously in that only one inversion pulse is applied for the entire data collection period. The contrast is determined by the effective TI, which is the user-selected TI plus the $G_{PE} = 0$ time:

$$TI_{effective} = TI + TR * N_{AQ} * N_{PE}/2 \qquad [5\text{-}2]$$

For T2 MP sequences, a series of rf pulses known as *driven equilibrium pulse train* is used. Three equally spaced rf pulses are applied with

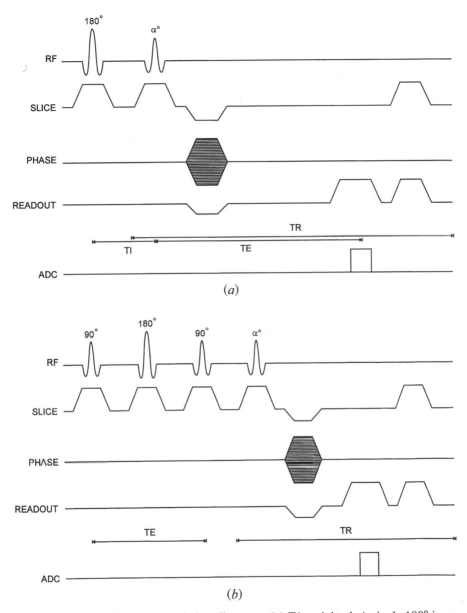

Figure 5-11. 2D-MP sequence timing diagrams. (*a*) T1-weighted. A single 180° inversion rf pulse is applied per scan. This inversion provides significant T1 weighting to **M**. The *TR* time period is executed for the desired N_{AQ} and N_{PE}; (*b*) T2-weighted. A 90°—180°—90° rf pulse train is applied prior to the data collection scheme. The first two pulses produce T2 weighting to **M** which is restored to the longitudinal direction by the final pulse prior to the data collection.

amplitudes $90°$-τ-$180°$-τ-$90°$ (Figure 5-11b). The first two pulses generate a spin echo and produce T2 weighting to the transverse magnetization. The third pulse rotates this magnetization into the longitudinal direction, producing changes in **M** based on the T2 relaxation times and the interpulse spacing τ. Use of a centric ordered data collection produces T2-weighted images with good contrast.

5.5 ECHO PLANAR IMAGING SEQUENCES

A second type of non-steady-state measurement technique, echo planar imaging (EPI), has a novel method for data collection. EPI sequences are characterized by a series of gradient reversals in the readout direction. Each reversal produces a gradient echo with the second half of one readout period being rephased by the first half of the subsequent readout period. The gradient reversals are performed very rapidly, allowing echo planar images to be acquired in 100–200 ms. Two types of schemes are used to phase encode each gradient echo. The constant phase-encoding method applies the phase-encoding gradient continuously throughout the readout period. A preparatory phase-encoding pulse is applied, then each echo is acquired with a different amount of total phase accumulation; that is, k space is sampled in a continuous and sinusoidal fashion (Figure 5-12a). Alternately, a "blipped" phase-encoding technique applies a small amplitude G_{PE} pulse prior to each sampling period. No phase-encoding gradient is applied during signal detection so that the phase encoding for each echo is constant (Figure 5-12b). The raw data matrix is acquired in a rectilinear, zig-zag fashion.

Two data collection schemes are used in EPI sequences: single shot and segmented or multishot. Single shot techniques acquire all phase encoding steps following a single excitation pulse. Since only one rf pulse is applied per slice position, each image can be acquired with an "infinite" *TR*. Special gradient amplifiers may be required for single-shot EPI imaging because of the rapid switching necessary to acquire all the echoes. Segmented techniques acquire a subset of phase-encoding steps following each excitation pulse. A segmented loop structure with multiple excitation pulses is used to acquire all phase-encoding steps. Segmented EPI can often be performed with standard imaging gradients.

The contrast in EPI images is determined by the *TE* for the echo acquired when the total $G_{PE} = 0$. Each echo is acquired at a different *TE* similar to echo train spin echo sequences, so the the *TE* in the image

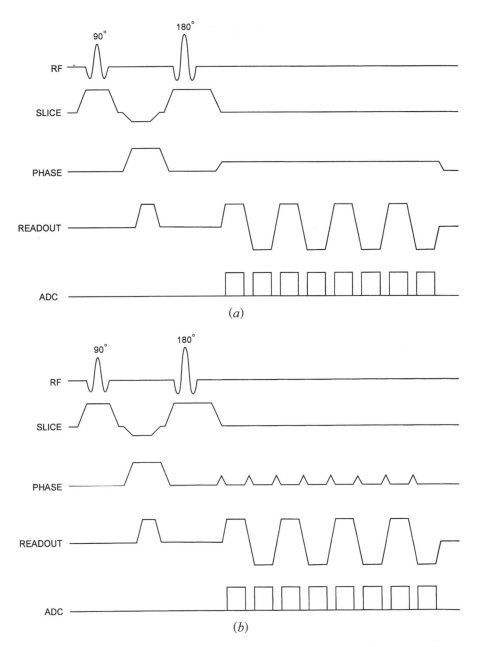

Figure 5-12. Echo planar imaging sequence timing diagrams. A spin echo excitation scheme and an echo train length of 8 are illustrated. (*a*) Constant phase encoding. The phase-encoding gradient is on for the entire data collection period. Each data point of each echo has a unique amount of G_{PE} amplitude. (*b*) Blipped phase encoding. The phase encoding gradient is incrementally applied prior to detection of cach echo. Each echo has a different amount of G_{PE}, but each data point within the echo has the same amount of G_{PE}.

is referred to as an effective *TE*. Variations in contrast for EPI sequences are achieved using preparatory pulses applied prior to the readout period. T1-weighted images are produced using a 180° inversion rf pulse prior to the excitation pulse. T2-weighted images can be obtained using a 90°–180° pair of pulses to produce a spin echo. Spoiled gradient echo EPI sequences use no preparatory pulse.

CHAPTER 6

Measurement Parameters and Image Contrast

Many MRI scan parameters can be adjusted by the operator through the user-interface software. These parameters affect not only the spatial resolution but also the inherent signal-to-noise (S/N) of the image and the intensity differences or contrast between adjacent tissues in the region of interest. One approach to categorizing the large number of these parameters is by their effect on the final image. *Intrinsic* parameters modify the inherent signal produced by a volume element of tissue (voxel). These parameters are most sensitive to the characteristic tissue properties that are the response to the measurement procedure. Intrinsic parameters affect only the signal producing portion of the image, which is normally patient anatomy and not background air. *Extrinsic* parameters influence the mechanics of data collection (e.g., voxel size) or other factors external to the tissue. Many of these parameters are dictated by the particular choice of pulse sequence used for the measurement. Extrinsic parameters typically affect the spatial resolution or general background noise levels in the final image.

6.1 INTRINSIC PARAMETERS

Repetition time, *TR*, measured in ms, is the time between successive rf excitation pulses applied to a given volume of tissue. In conjunction with the excitation angle (see following), *TR* determines the amount of T1 weighting contributing to the image contrast. If all other factors are equal, longer *TR* allows more time for the rf excitation energy to be dissipated by the protons through spin-lattice relaxation, producing images with less T1 weighting (Figure 6-1). For a multislice loop, *TR* limits the number of slices that can be acquired during the measurement.

Echo time, TE, measured in ms, is the time between the excitation pulse and the echo (signal) maximum. It determines the amount of T2

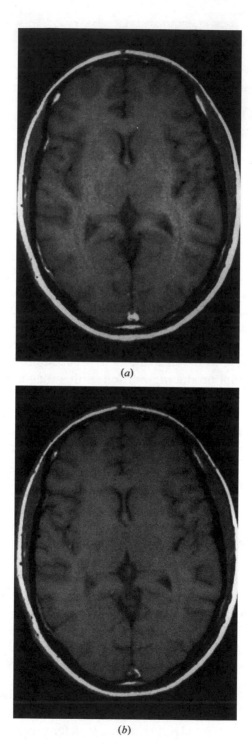

(a)

(b)

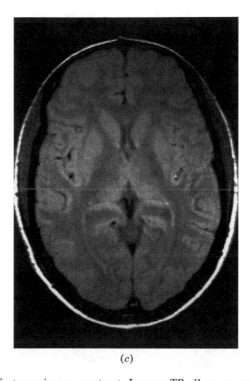

(*c*)

Figure 6-1. *TR* effects on image contrast. Longer *TR* allows more time for T1 relaxation and produces more signal from tissues with long T1 values. Other measurement parameters are: pulse sequence, spin echo; *TE*, 15 ms; excitation angle, 90°; acquisition matrix, 256 phase encoding steps, 256 readout data points; FOV, 230 × 230 mm²; acquisitions: *1*; slice thickness, 5mm. (*a*) *TR* of 350 ms; (*b*) *TR* of 650 ms; (*c*) *TR* of 2500 ms. Note reversal of contrast between gray matter and white matter in (*c*) compared to (*a*).

weighting for spin echo images (Figure 6-2). For gradient echo images, *TE* determines the amount of T2* weighting and the ratio of fat and water signal contributions (see Figure 2-5). Longer *TE* allows more time for proton dephasing and produces lower signal amplitudes. In echo train spin echo and echo planar sequences, *TE* is considered to be an effective *TE* since all echoes used in image reconstruction are not acquired at the same echo time.

Inversion time, *TI*, measured in ms, is the time between the 180° inversion pulse and the imaging excitation pulse. *TI* is used in inversion recovery (IR), echo train IR, and T1 magnetization-prepared sequences, and determines the amount of time allowed for T1 relaxation following the inversion pulse. Short *TI* times allow minimum T1 relaxation, while long *TI* times allow significant T1 relaxation prior to the imaging ex-

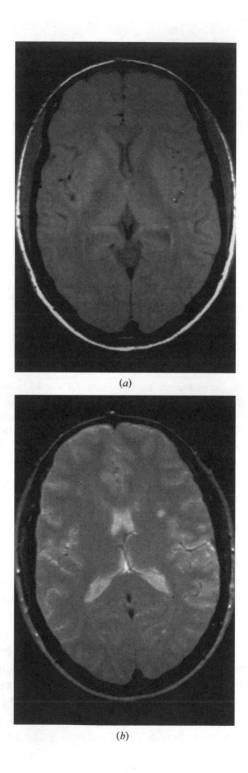

(a)

(b)

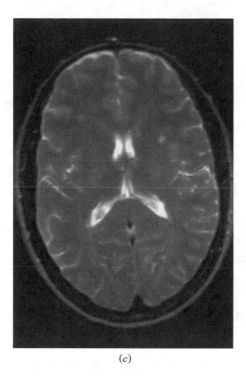

(c)

Figure 6-2. *TE* effects on image contrast. Longer *TE* allows more time for T2 relaxation and produces more signal from tissues with long T2 values. Other measurement parameters are: pulse sequence, spin echo; *TR*, 2500 ms; excitation angle, 90°; acquisition matrix, 256 phase encoding steps, 256 readout data points; *FOV*, 230 × 230 mm², acquisitions, *1*; slice thickness, 5 mm. (*a*) *TE* of 15 ms; (*b*) *TE* of 60 ms; (*c*) *TE* of 120 ms. Note bright signal from cerebrospinal fluid (CSF) in (*c*) compared to (*a*).

citation pulse. Proper choice of *TI* enables signal suppression of tissues based on their T1 relaxation times (Figure 6-3).

Echo train length (also known as the turbo factor) is the number of echoes (number of phase encoding steps) following an excitation pulse that is used to create an image. The echo train length is used in echo train spin echo and echo train inversion recovery sequences. Longer echo train lengths allow shorter scan times through more efficient data collection. The slice loop (minimum *TR* per slice) is longer with longer echo train lengths, producing greater signal attenuation through T2 relaxation as well as requiring longer slice loops. The number of phase encoding steps for the measurement is a multiple of the echo train length.

Echo spacing, measured in ms, and used in echo train spin echo and echo train inversion recovery sequences, is the time between each echo

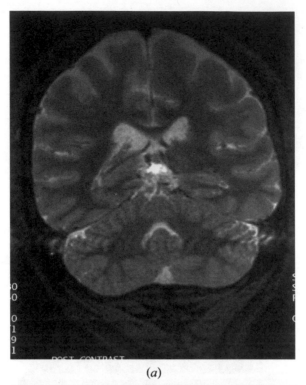

(a)

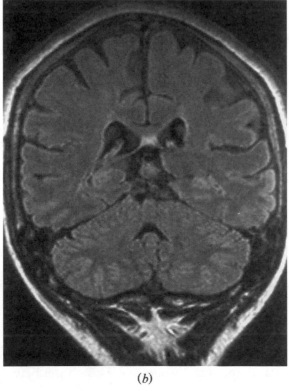

(b)

of the echo train. Longer echo spacing allows more time for T2 relaxation between each echo. Shorter echo spacing reduces the slice loop.

Excitation angle, measured in degrees and also known as the *flip angle*, is the amount of rotation away from the equilibrium axis that **M** undergoes through rf absorption. If not variable under the operating software, the excitation angle is usually 90° in order to generate the maximum transverse magnetization. The excitation angle is also proportional to the amount of energy absorbed and the amount of signal produced by the protons. The excitation angle, together with *TR* and the T1 values for the individual tissues, determines the amount of T1 weighting present in an image. The excitation angle that produces the maximum signal from a tissue for a particular *TR* is known as the *Ernst angle*.

6.2 EXTRINSIC PARAMETERS

Slice thickness, *TH*, measured in mm, is the volume of tissue in the slice selection direction that absorbs the rf energy during irradiation. Variation in slice thickness is usually accomplished through changing the magnitude of G_{SS}. Thicker slices provide more signal per voxel whereas thinner slices produce less partial volume averaging.

Slice gap, measured in mm, is the space between adjacent slices. The slice gap may also be expressed as a fraction of the slice thickness, depending on the operating software. The slice gap allows the user to control the size of the total imaging volume by increasing or decreasing space between slices. The slice gap also allows a method to compensate for the imperfect rf excitation pulses. If the slices are closely spaced, excitation pulses applied to adjacent slice position partially overlap and excite the same region of tissue because the slice excitation profiles are not uniform. This situation is known as *crosstalk* (Figure 6-4). Due to the rapid pulse application, these regions of overlap become saturated

---

Figure 6-3. *TI* effects on image contrast. Longer *TI* allows more time for T1 relaxation following the inversion pulse. The choice of *TI* can cause signal suppression of different tissues. Other measurement parameters are: pulse sequence, echo train inversion recovery; echo train length, 7; *TR*, 5000 ms; *TE*, 29 ms; Acquisition matrix, 168 phase encoding steps, 256 readout data points with twofold readout oversampling; FOV, 150 mm PE × 200 mm RO; acquisitions, *1*; slice thickness, 3 mm. (*a*) *TI* of 140 ms—fat suppression (STIR); (*b*) *TI* of 2210 ms—CSF suppression (FLAIR).

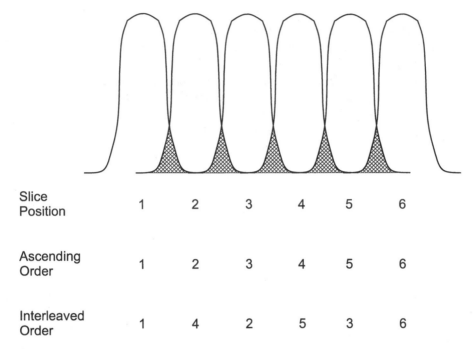

Slice Position	1	2	3	4	5	6
Ascending Order	1	2	3	4	5	6
Interleaved Order	1	4	2	5	3	6

Figure 6-4. Excitation order and crosstalk. If the slice gap is too small, then the bases of adjacent slices overlaps (shaded regions). Tissues located in this overlap region experience rf pulses from both slices and become saturated. This is called *crosstalk* and causes reduced signal from these regions. The order of slice excitation also determines the contribution of crosstalk to the image intensity. Sequential ordering of excitation (second row) acquires data from adjacent slice positions in successive time periods. Interleaved ordering (third row) acquires data from every other slice position first, then acquires data from the intermediate positions. This will minimize the effects of crosstalk between slices.

and contribute little to the detected signal. The slice gap allows space between adjacent slice positions and reduces the extent of crosstalk for the measurement.

Excitation order refers to the temporal order in which slices are excited during the measurement. Two ordering schemes are typically used (see Figure 6-4). Sequential ordering excites adjacent slice positions in successive time periods. This approach is preferred when relative timing of adjacent slices is critical, such as for electrocardiogram-triggered studies of the heart (see Chapter 9). Interleaved ordering excites alternate slices in successive time periods. Interleaved ordering allows the maximum amount of time for relaxation of the overlap region prior to the second excitation pulse. The effects of crosstalk are also reduced for all slices as much as possible. Arbitrary ordering may also be performed if allowed by the operating software.

The number of partitions, N_{PART}, is used in 3D volume studies and corresponds to the number of slices into which the excited volume is divided. The slices have signal derived from the total excited volume and are contiguous. The effective slice thickness is the volume excited (thickness) divided by N_{PART}. The scan time for a 3D sequence is linearly proportional to N_{PART} (equation [4-8]).

Field of view, FOV, measured in mm^2, specifies the area from which the MR signals are accurately sampled. The FOV may be specified separately for the readout and phase encoding directions (anisotropic or rectangular FOV), or it may be listed as a single number (isotropic or square FOV). Decreasing the FOV is accomplished by increasing the corresponding gradient amplitude. Increasing spatial resolution is achieved by decreasing the FOV, which decreases the voxel size at the expense of S/N.

The *acquisition matrix* (N_{PE}, N_{RO}) defines the raw data sampling grid used for the measurement of the base image. It consists of two numbers: One specifies the number of phase encoding steps (N_{PE}) and the other specifies the number of readout sampling data points (N_{RO}). Different manufacturers have conventions regarding which number is specified first. The acquisition matrix divides the FOV into individual areas which, together with the slice thickness, define the voxel size. Increased spatial resolution may be obtained by using larger acquisition matrices to produce smaller voxels. Data acquired beyond that necessary for defining the image FOV is referred to as *oversampling* and is used to reduce the presence of high frequency aliasing artifacts (see Chapter 8).

The *image matrix*, a, consists of the number of rows and columns of the image. Image matrices are usually square with equal numbers of rows and columns. Identification of row and column to readout and phase encoding directions is controlled through the operating software.

The number of acquisitions, N_{AQ}, (also known as N_{EX}, the number of excitation pulses) is the number of times the signal from a given slice for a given phase encoding amplitude is measured and added together for signal averaging. Depending on the operating software, all acquisitions may be performed at each phase encoding amplitude for a slice, or the entire set of phase encoding amplitudes may be measured for each slice before performing the second acquisition for any slice. The S/N ratio is proportional to the square root of N_{AQ} while the measurement time is proportional to N_{AQ}.

The receiver bandwidth BW_{REC}, measured in Hz, is the maximum frequency (Nyquist frequency) that can be accurately digitized. The Nyquist frequency depends on the sampling time and N_{RO}. The receiver bandwidth may also be expressed as the total bandwidth over the entire *FOV* or as the bandwidth per pixel, depending on the particular convention. Lower BW_{REC} improves the S/N at the expense of potentially larger chemical shift artifacts (see Chapter 8).

6.3 PARAMETER TRADEOFFS

Three criteria are used for determining a "good" measurement protocol: sufficient spatial resolution to resolve the underlying anatomy, reasonable signal-difference-to-noise (termed contrast-to-noise) ratio between tissues, and an acceptable measurement time. In general, these three criteria contradict one another, and the difficulty in protocol optimization is to obtain the proper balance between them. In addition, optimal parameters for one set of tissues may or may not be optimal for another set of tissues. Finally, while each parameter can be specified separately, they are not completely independent. For example, *TE* must be less than *TR*. The following formulas can provide guidance on the tradeoff of one parameter versus another for S/N or image intensity. Tables 6-1 and 6-2 also summarize the parameter changes and their effects on spatial resolution, S/N, and measurement time.

6.3.1 Extrinsic Variables

Standard 2D Imaging Acquisition:

$$\text{S/N}_{2D} = K(TH) \left(\frac{FOV_{RO}}{N_{RO}} \right) \left(\frac{FOV_{PE}}{N_{PE}} \right) \sqrt{\frac{N_{AQ}N_{RO}N_{PE}}{BW_{REC}}} \qquad [6\text{-}1]$$

Standard 3D Imaging Acquisition:

$$\text{S/N}_{3D} = K \left(\frac{TH}{N_{PART}} \right) \left(\frac{FOV_{RO}}{N_{RO}} \right) \left(\frac{FOV_{PE}}{N_{PE}} \right) \sqrt{\frac{N_{AQ}N_{RO}N_{PE}N_{PART}}{BW_{REC}}}$$

$$[6\text{-}2]$$

Equations [6-1] and [6-2] assume uniform tissue content and relaxation behavior throughout the excited volume. *K* contains constants and terms based on the intrinsic parameters. The terms in parentheses represent voxel dimensions and the square root term relates to noise con-

Table 6-1   Measurement Effects—Extrinsic Parameters

Parameter	Direction of Change	Effect on Spatial Resolution	Effect on S/N Ratio	Effect on Scan Time
TH	Increase	Decrease, linear	Increase, linear	None
N_{PART}	Increase	Increase, linear	Decrease, square root	Increase, linear
FOV_{RO}	Increase	Decrease, linear	Increase, linear	None
FOV_{PE}	Increase	Decrease, linear	Increase, linear	None
N_{RO}	Increase	Increase, linear	Decrease, square root	None
N_{PE}	Increase	Increase, linear	Decrease, square root	Increase, linear
N_{AQ}	Increase	None	Increase, square root	Increase, linear
BW_{REC}	Increase	None	Decrease, square root	None

tributions to the final measured signal. These equations may be used to estimate S/N changes for combinations of parameter changes. For example, the S/N changes in a linear manner with variation in slice thickness, but changes linearly with the square root of N_{AQ}. A twofold reduction in slice thickness may be offset by a fourfold increase in N_{AQ}.

6.3.2   Intrinsic Variables

Standard Single Spin Echo Signal Intensity

$$I_{SE} = N * K' * \exp(-TE/T2) * [1 - 2 \exp(-(TR - TE/2)/T1)$$

$$+ \exp(-TR/T1)] \qquad [6\text{-}3]$$

Table 6-2   Measurement Effects—Intrinsic Parameters

Parameter	Direction of Change	Effect on Spatial Resolution	Effect on S/N Ratio	Effect on Scan Time
TR	Increase	None	Increase	Increase, linear
TE	Increase	None	Decrease	None
Excitation angle α	Increase	None	Increase for Long TR Decrease for Short TR	None

Standard Inversion Recovery Signal Intensity

$$I_{IR} = N * K' * \exp(-TE/T2) * [1 - 2 \exp(-TI/T1)$$
$$+ 2 \exp(-(TR - TE/2)/T1) - \exp(-TR/T1)] \qquad [6\text{-}4]$$

Standard Spoiled Gradient Echo Signal Intensity

$$I_{SGE} = N * K' * \exp(-TE/T2^*) * \frac{\sin \alpha * (1 - \exp(-TR/T1))}{1 - \cos \alpha * \exp(-TR/T1)} \qquad [6\text{-}5]$$

Equations [6-3], [6-4], and [6-5] assume exact rf pulses of the desired flip angle. For the spin echo and inversion recovery equations, the excitation angle is assumed to be 90°. For the spoiled gradient echo equation, the excitation angle is α. K' contains constants and terms based on the extrinsic parameters and N is the number of protons per unit volume being excited.

CHAPTER 7

Additional Sequence Modifications

Chapter 5 presented the concept of a pulse sequence and described several classes of pulse sequences. The rf and gradient pulses were applied in very precisely defined ways to uniformly affect the signal intensity from all the protons within the volume of measured tissue. Additional rf excitation pulses may be added to any of these sequences to manipulate the net magnetization $\mathbf{M}$ for some of the tissue within the imaging volume and differentially affect its contribution to the detected signal. Three basic types of rf pulses may be added: frequency-selective pulses applied in conjunction with a gradient (spatial presaturation), frequency-selective pulses applied in the absence of a gradient (magnetization transfer suppression, fat saturation), and a series of rectangular, nonselective pulses (composite pulses). In all of these cases, additional time within the slice loop is required to implement the pulses. This reduces the maximum number of slices possible for a given TR when a multislice loop structure is used. In addition, the additional rf pulse(s) increases the total rf power deposition to the patient. Limitations due to the specific rate of rf energy absorption (SAR) (see Chapter 13) may be required, particularly for spin echo-based sequences using short TR.

7.1 SPATIAL PRESATURATION

Spatially localized presaturation pulses are frequency-selective rf pulses applied in conjunction with a gradient pulse that are used to suppress undesired signals from tissues within the imaging volume. They are often used for the suppression of artifactual signal from peristaltic and respiratory motion in lumbar spine imaging. Spatial presaturation pulses are also used to reduce blood flow artifacts from the aorta or inferior vena cava in abdominal imaging by saturating the blood before it enters the imaging volume. These types of pulses are also used to produce a tag for tracking portal blood flow.

Presaturation pulses are usually applied prior to the imaging slice pulses during sequence execution. They may be applied once per slice loop or once per *TR* time period. Due to their rapid occurrence, the presaturation pulses saturate the selected tissue so that its steady state net magnetization is much smaller than the net magnetization for the remaining tissue of the slice. In addition, spoiler gradients are applied to dephase any transverse magnetization following the presaturation pulse. The result is that the signal from the presaturated region is significantly less than the signal from the nonpresaturated tissue (Figure 7-1).

In addition to the problems regarding slice loop times and rf power deposition previously mentioned, spatial presaturation pulses will not remove all signal from the selected tissue. The saturated tissue experiences T1 relaxation during the time between the presaturation pulse and the imaging excitation pulse so that longitudinal magnetization is present within the presaturated region at the time the slice excitation pulse is applied. This generates signal from the saturated region that may have significant amplitude, depending on the particular *TR* for the measurement and the tissue T1 values. The amount of apparent signal suppression depends on the amount of signal produced in the saturated region relative to the signal produced in the unsaturated region.

7.2   FAT SATURATION

Normal MR imaging methods visualize protons from both water and fat molecules within the tissue. One method to selectively visualize only the tissue water is *fat saturation*. As mentioned in Chapter 2, fat and water have a chemical shift difference of approximately 3.5 ppm to their resonant frequencies. Fat saturation applies a narrow bandwidth rf pulse centered at the fat resonant frequency in the absence of a gradient. The resulting transverse magnetization is then dephased by spoiler gradients. A standard imaging sequence may then be performed, which produces images from the water protons within the slice (Figure 7-2a). The saturation pulse may be applied prior to every slice excitation pulse or once every phase encoding step. The signal suppression mechanism is similar to that of spatial presaturation described previously, in that minimal net magnetization from the fat is present at the time of the excitation pulse for the slice.

Fat saturation has two main advantages over STIR imaging for fat suppression (see Chapter 5). It may be used with any type of imaging

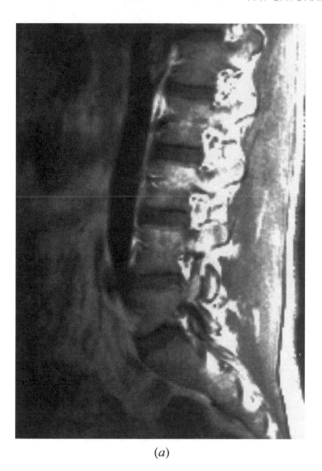

(*a*)

Figure 7-1. Application of a spatial presaturation pulse to moving tissue will suppress signal from that tissue. Measurement parameters are: pulse sequence, spin echo; *TR*, 500 ms; *TE*, 15 ms; excitation angle, 90°; acquisition matrix, 192 phase encoding steps, 256 readout data points with 2× frequency oversampling; FOV, 210 mm PE × 280 mm RO; acquisitions, 3; slice thickness, 4 mm. (*a*) No presaturation pulse; (*b*) Coronal spatial presaturation pulse, suppressing anterior abdominal tissue. *Illustration continued on following page.*

sequence. T1 fat saturation sequences may also be used with T1 contrast agents since the contrast agent shortens the T1 relaxation times of only the water protons (see Chapter 14). The T1 reduction enables the enhanced tissues to generate significant signal while the fat signal remains minimal in the presence or absence of the contrast agent. However, three potential problems are inherent with fat saturation, in addition to the problems of increased slice loop time and rf power deposition. One is that there will be magnetization transfer suppression (see following) of

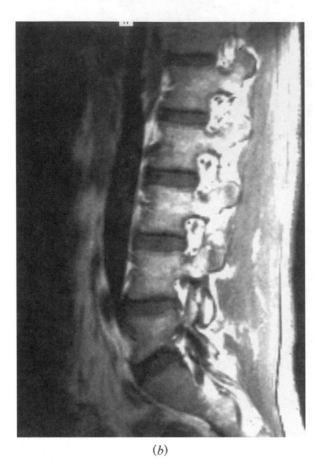

(*b*)

Figure 7-1. (*Continued*)

the water protons by the saturation pulse. The second problem is that the fat protons undergo T1 relaxation during the time between the saturation pulse and the imaging pulses and contribute to the detected signal. As the fat signal approaches the water signal in amplitude, the contrast between the fat and water tissues is reduced. Finally, fat saturation is particularly sensitive to the magnetic field homogeneity. The exact frequency difference between fat and water protons depends upon the magnetic field that a voxel experiences. If the homogeneity is not uniform throughout the imaging volume, the center frequency of the saturation pulse will be off-resonance for some of the fat and will not suppress it. In some cases, the water protons may be saturated rather than the fat protons (Figure 7-2*b*). For this reason, optimization of the field homogeneity to the specific patient prior to applying a fat saturation pulse is advisable.

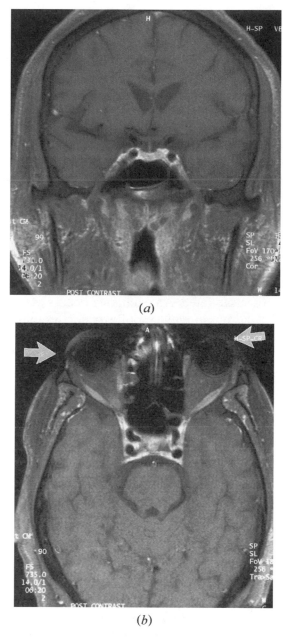

(a)

(b)

Figure 7-2. Frequency-selective saturation (fatsat) pulse is applied to suppress signal from fat protons. (a) With a homogeneous magnetic field, the suppression of fat is uniform throughout the slice; (b) With a nonhomogeneous magnetic field, the saturation pulse suppresses fat in one region of the image and water in other regions (arrows). Measurement parameters are: pulse sequence, spin echo; TR, 735 ms; TE, 14 ms; excitation angle, 90°; matrix, 256 phase encoding steps, 512 readout data points with twofold frequency oversampling; FOV, 170 × 170 mm²; acquisitions, 2; slice thickness, 4 mm.

7.3 MAGNETIZATION TRANSFER SUPPRESSION

Another suppression technique similar in hardware implementation to fat saturation is magnetization transfer suppression, which is used to selectively irradiate water protons that have very short T2 values. Water within a tissue is either mobile (freely moving) or bound (adsorbed to macromolecules). The bound fraction water protons have a very short T2 due to the rapid dephasing they undergo. The resonance peak is very broad and normally does not contribute significantly to the measured signal. The mobile water molecules have a much longer T2 and a narrow resonance peak. These two resonances are superimposed at the same center frequency (Figure 7-3).

Magnetization transfer suppression is accomplished using a narrow bandwidth saturation pulse known as a magnetization transfer (MT) pulse centered 1–10 kHz away from the central water frequency applied in the absence of a gradient. The bound water protons are selectively irradiated and become saturated. An exchange occurs between the bound water protons and the unsaturated mobile water protons that transfers the saturation to the mobile fraction protons causing a loss of steady state magnetization and reducing the signal from the mobile fraction protons. This process is called magnetization transfer suppression. Contrast is enhanced between tissues that undergo magnetization transfer (water-containing tissues) and those that do not (fat-containing tissues). Magnetization transfer pulses may be used in spin echo or gradient echo sequences to produce additional signal suppression of tissue water.

Magnetization transfer suppression is most often used for suppression of normal tissue water in studies where normal tissue is of little interest. Two examples illustrate this. Time-of-flight MR angiography (see Chapter 10) is a technique for visualizing blood flow within the vascular network. Suppression of the normal brain tissue water using magnetization transfer pulses enables smaller vessels to be distinguished (Figure 7-4). The other application of magnetization transfer is T1 studies following the administration of a contrast agent. T1 contrast agents shorten the T1 relaxation time for tissues where the agent is located (see Chapter 14). Comparison of images acquired pre- and post-contrast administration enable determination of the agent dispersal. Use of a magnetization transfer pulse during the postcontrast measurement reduces the signal from the unenhanced tissues, providing greater contrast with the enhanced tissue (Figure 7-5).

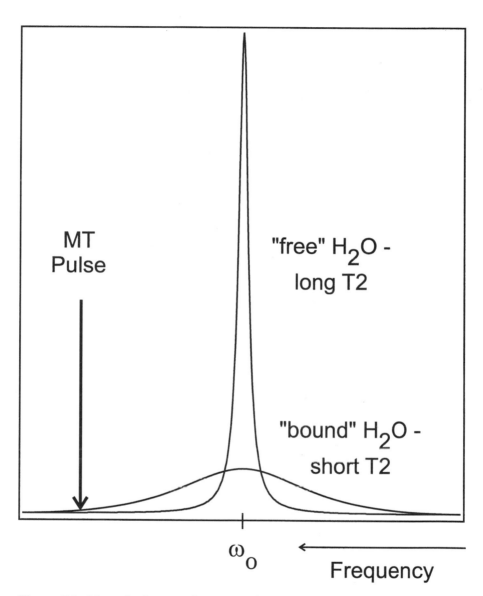

Figure 7-3. Magnetization transfer suppression. Mobile of "free" tissue water has protons with long T2 values and produces a narrow resonance peak. Water adsorbed or "bound" to macromolecules has protons with short T2 values and produces a wide resonance peak normally not visualized in an image. Both types of water protons have the same resonant frequency. The magnetization transfer rf pulse is applied off-resonance to saturate the bound water protons. Exchange between the bound and free water transfers the saturation to the free water protons, reducing signal intensity from the free water.

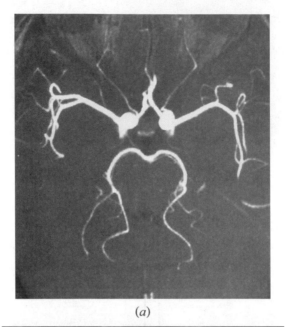

(a)

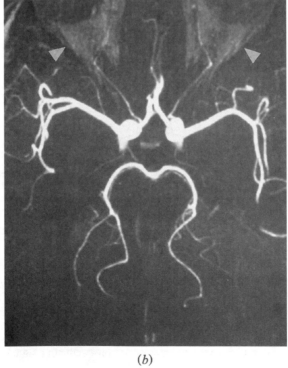

(b)

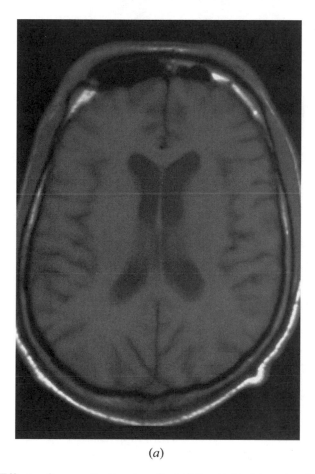

(*a*)

Figure 7-5. Effects of magnetization transfer in T1-weighted imaging following contrast administration. Application of MT pulse suppresses background signal from normal matter, enabling better visualization of contrast-enhanced tissues such as tumors or vascular structures. Measurement parameters are: pulse sequence, spin echo; *TR*, 560 ms; *TE*, 15 ms; excitation angle, 90°; acquisition matrix, 192 phase encoding steps, 256 readout data points with twofold readout oversampling; *FOV*, 173 mm PE × 230 mm RO; acquisitions, 1; slice thickness, 6 mm. (*a*) No MT pulse; (*b*) MT pulse. *Illustration continued on following page.*

◄――

Figure 7-4. Effects of magnetization transfer in 3-D MR angiography. Application of MT pulse suppressed background signal from gray and white matter, enabling better visualization of blood vessels. An apparent increase in signal from suborbital fat is observed (arrows). Measurement parameters are: pulse sequence, 3D refocused gradient echo, postexcitation; *TR*, 42 ms; *TE*, 7 ms; excitation angle, 25°; acquisition matrix, 192 phase encoding steps, 512 readout data points with twofold readout oversampling; *FOV*, 201 mm PE × 230 mm RO; acquisitions, 1; effective slice thickness, 0.78 mm. (*a*) No MT pulse; (*b*) MT pulse.

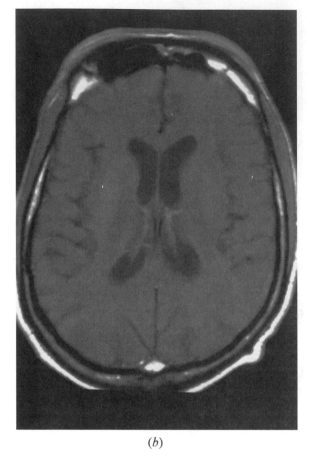

(*b*)

Figure 7-5. (*Continued*)

7.4 COMPOSITE PULSES

A composite rf pulse is a series of closely spaced rf pulses applied over a short time period that affect the protons life a single pulse. The pulse amplitudes for each rf pulse typically form a binomial progression (e.g., 11, 121, 1331), with the effective flip angle being the sum of the individual flip angles. The timing between the pulses allows protons with different resonant frequencies to cycle in phase and undergo different effects from each pulse (Figure 7-6). The individual pulses may be nonselective (rectangular) or frequency selective, resulting in a composite pulse of the same character. In general, composite pulses require less

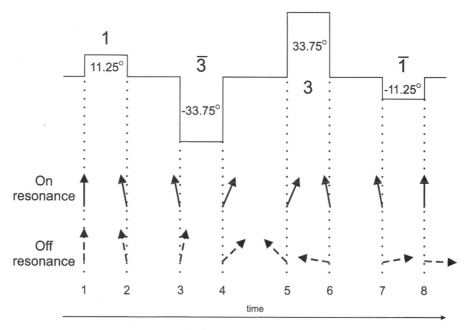

Figure 7-6. Composite pulse. A $\overline{1}33\overline{1}$ composite pulse is shown with a total excitation angle of 90°. A rotating frame corresponding to the on-resonant frequency is assumed. Prior to the first rf pulse (1), both on-resonance (solid arrow) and off-resonance (dashed arrow) protons are unexcited. At the end of the first rf pulse (2), both will be excited 11.25°. Because of the difference in resonant frequencies, the off resonant protons become out of phase. The time for the second rf pulse (3) is chosen so that the off-resonance protons are exactly 180° out of phase. At the end of the second rf pulse (4), the off-resonance protons are excited −45° while the on-resonance protons are excited −22.5°. The delay between the second and third rf pulses is chosen so that the off-resonance protons are 180° out of phase with the on-resonance proton (5). A similar delay is chosen between the third and fourth rf pulses (6,7). At the end of the fourth rf pulse (8), the on-resonance protons are at 0° (unexcited), while the off-resonance protons are rotated 90°.

transmitter power than single rf pulses for the same flip angle because of the short duration of the individual pulses.

Composite pulses can be used for general slice excitation, but the most common application is for fat suppression. A composite pulse is used that excites the fat protons and leaves the water protons unexcited. Spoiler gradients may be applied to dephase the fat transverse magnetization. Application of a standard imaging pulse or pulse produces signal from only the tissue water. Alternately, a composite pulse can be used to selectively excite the water protons by changing the relative polarity of the individual pulses. Known as water excitation, gradient spoiling is not necessary for elimination of the fat signal. Composite pulses are very sensitive to field homogeneity since differences in the resonant frequency change the cycling time for fat relative to water. Poor homogeneity causes undesired excitation and/or incomplete suppression. For this reason, optimization of the field homogeneity to each patient is advisable.

CHAPTER 8

Artifacts

Artifacts in MR images refer to pixels that do not faithfully represent the anatomy being studied. The general appearance of the images is that the underlying anatomy is visualized but spurious signals are present that do not correspond to actual tissue at that location. The artifacts may or may not be easily discernible from normal anatomy, particularly since they may be of low intensity and may or may not be reproducible. Artifacts can be categorized in many ways; one approach divides them into three groups according to the cause of the signal misregistration. The first group is a consequence of motion of patient tissue during the measurement. This includes both gross physical motion by the patient and blood flow. The second group is produced primarily as a result of the particular measurement technique and/or specific measurement parameters. The final group of artifacts is generated by a malfunction of the MR scanner during data collection or from a source external to the patient or scanner.

8.1 MOTION ARTIFACTS

Motion artifacts occur as a result of movement of tissue during the data acquisition period. They are manifest as signal misregistrations in the phase-encoding direction, though the specific appearance of the artifact depends on the nature of the motion and the particular measurement. Motion artifacts are caused by tissue that is excited at one location producing signals that are mapped to a different location during detection. As mentioned in Chapter 4, the typical MRI scan excites and detects signal from a tissue volume multiple times with the phase-encoding gradient changing amplitude between each step. The assumption is made that any measured signal intensity variations from one measurement to the next are as a result of G_{PE} only. When tissue moves, the protons are at a different location at the time of detection and experience a different G_{RO} gradient amplitude, producing a different frequency and phase for that measurement. The Fourier transformation mismaps these protons to an incorrect location along the phase-encoding direction in the image. In general, many measurements are made in the production of an image, each with a different amount of motion contamination. The Fourier transformation of the entire set of measurements does not result in a unique set of frequencies and phases, but in multiple signals in the phase-encoding direction throughout the entire *FOV*. The misregistered signals occur along the phase-encoding direction rather than the readout direction because the encoding of phase by a gradient occurs prior to signal detection for the phase-encoding gradient while it occurs concurrent with signal detection for the readout gradient.

The sensitivity of a measurement to motion depends on the particular phase-encoding amplitude that is applied for the contaminated measurement. If the motion occurs during measurements with low amplitude G_{PE} (at the center of k space), then the misregistered signal possesses considerable amplitude and contributes substantially to the final image. If the motion occurs during measurements with high amplitude positive or negative G_{PE} (at the edges of k space), the detected signals have very little amplitude and generate minimal artifact.

Probably the most common motion artifact in MRI is due to blood flow. The artifact from blood flow is dependent on the nature of the flow and the flow direction relative to the slice orientation. Through-plane flow, flow that is perpendicular to the slice plane, typically produces a localized artifact in the image with a width equal to the vessel diameter and in line with the origin of the flow. If the flow is relatively periodic, then the artifact appears as "ghost" vessels at discrete points. This is often seen from blood flow in the aorta or inferior vena cava (IVC) in transverse slices of the abdomen (Figure 8-1). In-plane flow, flow parallel to the slice plane, produces a more global artifact, which can be seen in the aorta and IVC in coronal images. The vessel extends through the entire image field and thus the artifact affects all regions of the image. Flow of the cerebrospinal fluid in the brain and spinal canal are also problematic, and can produce analogous artifacts on T2-weighted images (Figure 8-2).

In abdominal or lumbar spine imaging, respiratory motion and peristalsis are the most common causes of severe artifactual signal. The movement of the abdomen during the data collection process produces multiple misregistration artifacts. If the respiration rate is constant, the ghost images are few in number or discrete and offset in the phase-encoding direction from the true image by an amount proportional to the respiration rate. If the respiration rate is variable, the ghost images

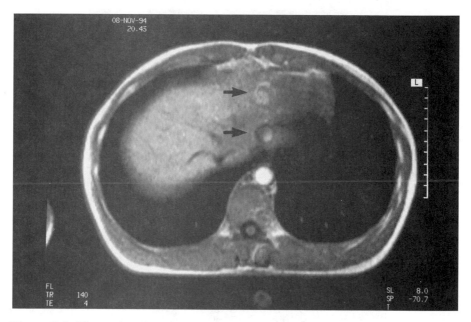

Figure 8-1. Flow misregistration artifact. Blood from the aorta will be misregistered as a "ghost" (arrows). Lesions in the left lobe of the liver may be obscured. Measurement parameters are: pulse sequence, spoiled gradient echo; *TR*, 140 ms; *TE*, 4 ms; acquisition matrix, 128 phase encoding steps, 256 readout data points with twofold oversampling; *FOV*, 350 × 350 mm²; acquisitions, 1; slice thickness, 8 mm; phase-encoding direction, A–P; readout direction, L–R.

are numerous and appear as a smearing of signal throughout the entire image (Figure 8-3*a*). For fast spin echo techniques, respiratory motion may show multiple lines or so-called venetian blinds superimposed over the image. The number and spacing of the lines corresponds to the number of segments in each rf pulse (Figure 8-3*b*). Peristalsis produces motion artifacts that are less distinct than those from respiratory motion. In most instances, a general blurring of the large and small bowel occurs and a layer of noise is superimposed over the entire image.

8.2   SEQUENCE/PROTOCOL-RELATED ARTIFACTS

A second class of artifacts results from the specific measurement process used to acquire the image. While the appearance of motion artifacts also depends on the particular measurement protocol, this group of artifacts is more sensitive to technical aspects of the particular pulse sequence

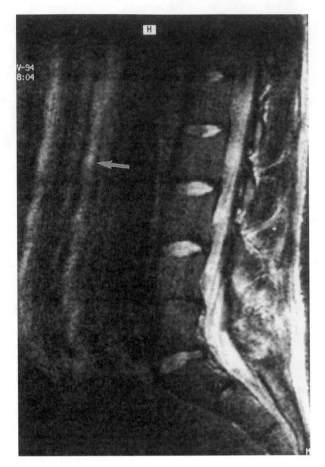

Figure 8-2. Flow misregistration artifact. Flowing CSF will be misregistered as a "ghost" canal (arrow). Measurement parameters are: pulse sequence, spin echo; *TR*, 2500 ms; *TE*, 90 ms; excitation angle, 90°; acquisition matrix, 192 phase encoding steps, 256 readout data points with 2× frequency oversampling; *FOV*, 210 mm PE × 280 mm RO; acquisitions, 1; slice thickness, 5 mm; phase-encoding direction, A–P; readout direction: H–F.

and method of data collection used. The origin of these artifacts is relatively constant over the course of the measurement and the resulting signal misregistrations are easily recognized when present.

8.2.1   Aliasing

The techniques used for spatial localization assign a unique frequency and phase to each location within the image. This is determined by the

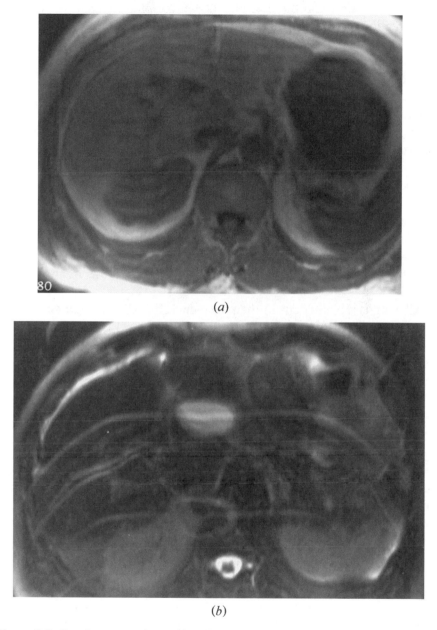

(*a*)

(*b*)

Figure 8-3. Respiratory motion artifact. Extraneous "ghost" images are generated due to motion of the abdominal wall during data acquisition. The number and severity of the ghosts depends on the *TR*, respiration rate, and the particular measurement technique. (*a*) Pulse sequence, spoiled gradient echo; *TR*, 140 ms; (*b*) Pulse sequence, echo train spin echo; *TR*, 5000 ms.

acquisition matrix and the desired *FOV* in the phase-encoding and read-out directions. A problem occurs when tissue outside the chosen *FOV* is excited. This can occur when a *FOV* smaller than the anatomical region is selected. The frequencies for this tissue exceed the Nyquist limit for the sampling conditions and are mapped to a lower frequency, a situation known as *high frequency aliasing* or *frequency wraparound* (Figure 8-4a). The technique used to overcome this is known as *frequency oversampling*, in which the number of readout data points is increased while maintaining the same sampling time and the same read-out gradient amplitude. This condition increases the Nyquist frequency for the measurement, according to equation [2-2]. Because G_{RO} is constant, the frequencies at the chosen *FOV* are unchanged, so that extraction of the central range of frequencies produce an image of the desired size and number of data points. For example, for a 256 * 256 matrix with twofold frequency oversampling, 512 data points are measured but only the central 256 data points are used to create the image (Figure 8-4b).

Aliasing can also occur in the phase encoding direction when protons outside the *FOV* are excited. These protons undergo phase changes corresponding to frequencies greater than can be accurately measured for the G_{PE} pulse duration (Nyquist limit). They are mapped via the Fourier transformation to a lower phase, in a manner analogous to the aliasing in the readout direction described earlier. Phase-encoding aliasing can only be eliminated by increasing the effective *FOV* in the phase-encoding direction. This may be accomplished either by reducing the change in gradient amplitude from one phase-encoding step to the next (increasing the *FOV*) or by increasing the number of phase changes (i.e., Nyquist frequency) while maintaining the same change in gradient amplitude, a technique known as *phase encoding oversampling*. Because more echoes are acquired, phase encoding oversampling will increase the total measurement time.

Figure 8-4. Effects of oversampling. (*a*) Without frequency oversampling, frequencies for the protons within the arms exceed the Nyquist limit and are aliased or incorrectly mapped into the image (arrows). Measurement parameters are: pulse sequence, spoiled gradient echo; *TR*, 140 ms; *TE*, 4 ms; excitation angle, 80°; acquisition matrix, 128 phase-encoding steps, 256 readout data points; *FOV*, 263 mm PE × 350 mm RO; acquisitions, 1; slice thickness, 8 mm; (*b*) Same as Figure 8-4a except with frequency oversampling. The frequencies for the protons within the arms are accurately measured

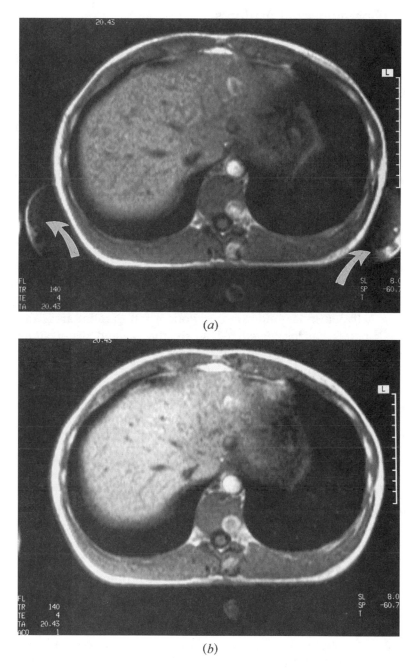

(a)

(b)

by increasing the number of readout data points measured during the same sampling
time while maintaining the same G_{RO}. Only frequencies corresponding to the selected
FOV are stored so that the arms are excluded from the final image. Measurement
parameters are same as (a) except 512 readout data points.

8.2.2 Chemical Shift Artifacts

Chemical-shift-based artifacts arise from the inherent 3.5 ppm frequency difference between fat and water protons under the influence of an external magnetic field as described in Chapter 2. Two static artifacts may be generated by this frequency difference. One is the chemical shift artifact, which is a misregistration of fat and water protons from a voxel that are mapped to different pixels. As described in Chapter 4, the detected signal from a voxel is mapped to a position based on its frequency according to equation [4-1], under the assumption that all protons within a voxel resonate at the same frequency. Due to the difference in molecular structure, fat protons have an intrinsically lower resonant frequency than water protons for the same external magnetic field. Fat protons within a voxel are affected by the same G_{RO} as the water protons but will be mapped to a lower frequency pixel in the readout direction. This misregistration is not noticeable in tissues with uniform fat–water content, but can be seen at the borders between tissues with significantly different fat–water content such as between disk and vertebrae in the spine or between kidney and retroperitoneal fat. Parallel areas of bright and dark pixels can be visualized where the fat and water signals superimpose and where they do not, respectively (Figure 8-5a). The number of pixels corresponding to the chemical shift artifact (CSA) depends upon the frequency difference in Hz between fat and water, the total receiver bandwidth, and the number of readout data points spanning the *FOV* (equation [8-1]):

$$CSA = \Delta\omega * N_{RO}/BW_{REC} \qquad [8\text{-}1]$$

At 1.5 T, the frequency difference is 220 Hz so that, for a sequence with a total receiver bandwidth of 20 kHz and $N_{RO} = 256$, the CSA will be 2.8 pixels. If a *FOV* of 350×350 mm^2 is used, this translates into a fat/water misregistration of 3.6 mm. For a sequence with a receiver bandwidth of 33 kHz, the CSA will be 1.7 pixels and a misregistration of 2.2 mm. Chemical shift artifacts are most prominent at 1.5 T, using

---

Figure 8-5. Chemical shift artifact. (*a*) Note alternate bands of light and dark (arrows) at the interface between the kidneys and retroperitoneal fat. Measurement parameters are pulse sequence, spin echo; receiver bandwidth 20 kHz; readout direction, L–R; (*b*) A complete misregistration of fat from the bone marrow of the skull (arrow). Measurement parameters are: pulse sequence, spin echo EPI; phase-encoding direction, A–P.

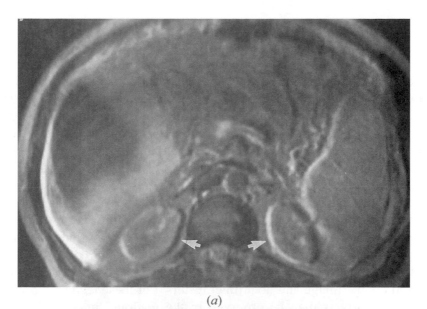

(*a*)

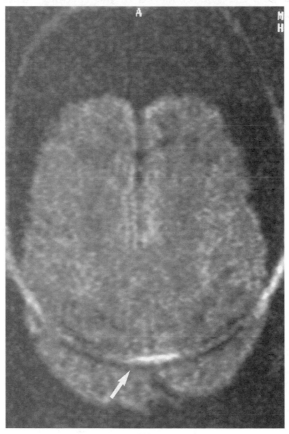

(*b*)

low or narrow receiver bandwidth sequences, and at fat–water tissue interfaces.

In theory, chemical shift artifacts are possible in all three directions (slice selection, phase encoding, and readout), since magnetic field variations (gradient pulses) are used for localization in all cases. In the slice selection direction, the rf pulse bandwidth and gradient amplitude are chosen to keep this at a minimum. In addition, because the slice selection direction is not directly visualized, any misregistration in this direction is difficult to discern. The appearance of the chemical shift artifact in the readout and phase-encoding directions depends on the particular pulse sequence. For routine imaging techniques such as spin echo, fast spin echo, or gradient echo, the phase-encoding process is reinitiated following each excitation pulse. The change in G_{PE} from one step to the next is constant so that fat and water protons located at the same position undergo equal amounts of phase change. They are mapped to the same location in the image and no artifact results. For these techniques, chemical shift artifacts may be observed in the readout direction, based on the specific criteria described previously. For echo planar imaging, the receiver bandwidth is very large (in excess of 100 kHz) so that fat and water frequencies are mapped to the same pixel. However, the phase-encoding process for the entire image occurs in a continuous fashion following one or two excitation pulses. Chemical shift artifacts will be observed in the phase-encoding direction and are very significant. Because the phase-encoding gradient amplitude is very low amplitude, the misregistration may be as much as 12–15 pixels (Figure 8-5*b*). Use of fat suppression techniques is necessary to minimize the artifact.

8.2.3 Phase Cancellation Artifact

The second artifact induced by the chemical shift difference is known as the *phase cancellation artifact* observed in out-of-phase gradient echo images. As shown in Figure 2-6, the fat protons cycle in phase relative to the water proton precession. For normal spin echo and fast spin echo sequences, this phase cycling is exactly reversed by the 180° rf pulse(s) so that the fat and water protons always contribute to the signal at the echo time, *TE*, with the same polarity; that is, the fat and water protons are described as "in phase" when the signal is detected regardless of the choice of *TE*. In gradient echo sequences, the phase cycling is not reversed and causes fat and water protons to contribute differently to the detected signal, depending on the particular *TE*. Voxels containing both fat and water have additional signal intensity variations in addition to those due to relaxation. For certain choices of *TE*, very little signal will be detected if the voxel has equal water and fat content such as those voxels located at tissue interfaces. This signal cancellation appears as a dark ring surrounding the tissue (Figure 8-6).

The *TE* values that generate this phase cancellation depend on the magnetic field strength, since the time for the phase cycling depends upon the resonant frequency difference $\Delta\omega_{fw}$ in Hz between fat and water:

$$TE_{inphase} = 1/\Delta\omega_{fw} \qquad [8\text{-}2]$$

At 1.0 T, the in-phase images occur at *TE*s of 6.7, 13.5, and 20 ms while at 1.5 T, the *TE* times are 4.5, 9, 13.5, and 18 ms. The out-of-phase *TE* times occur midway between the in-phase times. Out-of-phase images are often used to determine the amount of fat contribution to a voxel. The phase cancellation artifact observed using out-of-phase *TE* makes it difficult to assess the interface of tissues with different fat and water content. The phase cycling also affects the signal content of all tissues throughout the image. Unless there is specific reason for using an out-of-phase *TE* such as for the assessment of fatty infiltration in the liver or adrenal masses or to use very short *TR*, a *TE* corresponding to an in-phase relationship is preferable.

8.2.4 Truncation Artifacts

Truncation artifacts are produced by insufficient digital sampling of the echo. The most common instance of this condition occurs when data collection is terminated while significant signal is still being emitted by the protons, which can happen in T1-weighted imaging where there is high signal from fat at the edge of the region still present at the end of data collection. The Fourier transformation of this truncated data set produces a "ringing"-type of signal oscillation that emanates from the edge of the anatomy (Figure 8-7). Truncation artifacts can also occur if the echo is sampled in an asymmetrical fashion; that is, the echo is not sampled equally on both sides of the echo maximum (Figure 8-8). This type of data sampling is often used in very short *TE* sequences (<3 ms) to minimize the receiver bandwidth.

Reduction of truncation artifacts involves reducing the signal amplitude so that it is minimal at the end of the data collection period. This reduction can be achieved in two ways. One is to reduce the fat signal through fat suppression, either using a fat saturation pulse or using an inversion recovery technique. This approach changes the intrinsic image

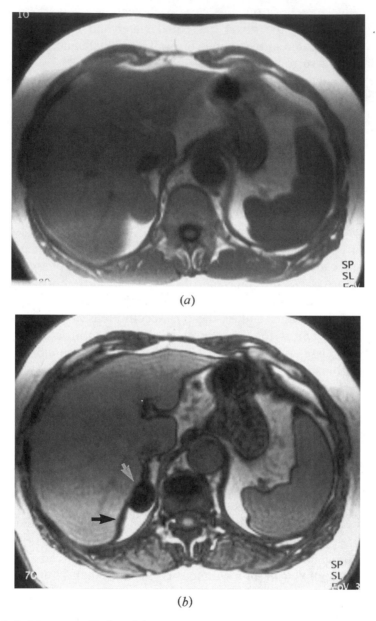

(a)

(b)

Figure 8-6. Phase cancellation. Other measurement parameters are: pulse sequence, 2D spoiled gradient echo; *TR*, 135 ms; excitation angle, 80°; acquisition matrix, 128 phase-encoding steps, 256 readout data points with 2× frequency oversampling; *FOV*, 306 mm PE × 350 mm RO; acquisitions, 1; slice thickness, 9 mm. (*a*) In-phase image (*TE* 4.5 ms). Fat and water protons have the same phase and contribute in the same fashion to the image contrast. (*b*) Out-of-phase image (*TE* 2.2 ms). Fat and water protons have opposite phases and contribute in opposite fashion to the image contrast. For voxels

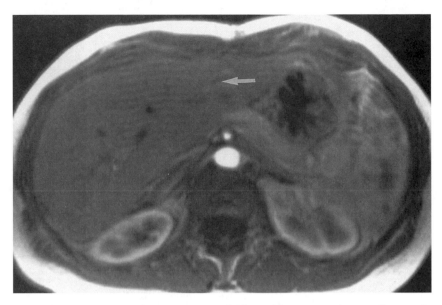

Figure 8-7. Truncation artifact. Image acquisition with asymmetric sampling produces a banding artifact (arrow), originating from the high signal of subcutaneous fat. Pulse sequence, spoiled gradient echo; *TR*, 170 ms; *TE*, 4 ms; excitation angle, 80°; acquisition matrix, 144 phase-encoding steps, 256 readout datapoints with twofold oversampling; *FOV*, 262 mm PE × 350 mm RO; acquisitions, 1.

contrast and may be unacceptable for the particular clinical application. The other method is to apply an apodization filter to the raw data prior to Fourier transformation. This numerical process forces the signal amplitude to zero at the end of the data collection period. Several types of apodization filters are available (e.g., Fermi, Gaussian, Hanning), each with different characteristics regarding the filter shape. Use of apodization filters improves the signal-to-noise ratio by removing high-frequency noise from the signal. However, excessive filtering eliminates high frequencies responsible for fine spatial resolution or edge definition so that blurring is possible. Asymmetric echo sampling may require more extensive filtering to reduce truncation artifacts. Acquiring the echo in a symmetric fashion reduces the amount of filtering necessary.

---

with equal amounts of fat and water, such as at the interface between liver and retroperitoneal fat, cancellation of signal occurs, producing a dark band (black arrow). Note the significant reduction in signal from the adrenal gland (white arrow), characteristic of an adenoma.

a.

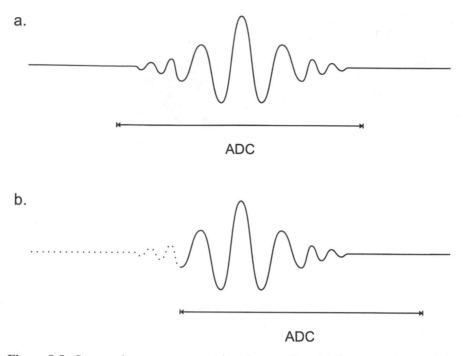

ADC

b.

ADC

Figure 8-8. Symmetric versus asymmetric echo sampling. (*a*) In symmetric sampling, the echo is formed midway through the sampling period so that both sides of the echo signal are measured equally. Filtering of the data can be performed in a symmetrical fashion. (*b*) In asymmetric sampling, the echo forms in the early portion of the sampling period. Significant signal is present when the sampling begins and filtering of the signal is difficult.

8.2.5 Coherence Artifacts

Coherence artifacts are a class of artifacts that can have a variable appearance, based on the particular measurement technique and how it is implemented on the scanner. They are produced by the rf pulses generating unwanted transverse magnetization that contributes to the detected signal. One coherence artifact is known as an FID artifact. As mentioned in Chapter 4, the rf excitation pulses are not uniform in profile. For instance, while most of the protons in a slice would experience a 180° excitation pulse, those located at the edges of the slice would experience a range of excitation angles, all less than 180°. The FID from these protons may still be producing significant signal when the desired echo signal is measured. Because the 180° rf pulse normally occurs after the phase encoding gradient during sequence execution, the induced signal will contribute identically during each ADC sampling period. The resulting artifact is a line of constant phase in the final image.

Another coherence artifact may be produced by the effects of the multiple rf excitation pulses on the protons. The spin echoes used to produce T1- and T2-weighted images are but two of several echoes generated by rf excitation pulses within an imaging sequence. For example, a series of 3 rf pulses such as a presaturation pulse and a 90°-180° pulse pair or a 90°-180°-180° pulse trio may generate 4 or 5 echoes. The timing and number of echoes depends on the exact spacing of the pulses (Figure 8-9). The amplitude of each echo depends on the excitation angle of the individual pulses and the particular tissues being measured. These "secondary" echoes contain all the frequency information of the so-called primary echoes normally used, but have different T1 and T2 weighting to the signals. Should these other echoes occur while the ADC is sampling the primary echoes, they will contribute to the final image. They may produce either line artifacts if not phase encoded, or an additional image if phase encoded (Figure 8-10). One of these echoes, the stimulated echo, is incorporated into the design of fast spin echo imaging techniques and in the volume selection in MR spectroscopy (Chapter 12).

Pulse sequences are usually designed with great care to minimize the contamination of the desired echo signals by the undesired echoes. When these undesired echoes form during the ADC sampling period due to the particular rf pulse timing, some form of coherence spoiling is used. Two approaches are used to dephase the transverse magnetization so that there is minimal coherence present from these secondary echoes. The most common method is to include additional gradient pulses applied at appropriate times during the pulse sequence, an approach known as *gradient spoiling*. These gradient pulses are usually of high amplitude and/or long duration. The time when these pulses are applied depends on which coherence is to be spoiled and what *TE* is chosen. Spoiler gradients applied following the 180° refocusing pulse reduce the FID artifact resulting from nonuniform rf excitation. Spoiler gradients following the data collection such as those used in spin echo sequences (see Figure 5-2) minimizes coherence contamination of the subsequent echoes. For many sequences, the duration of the spoiler gradient pulse may be 30–50% of the slice loop. Gradient spoiling may also use a series of amplitudes rather than a constant amplitude pulse in order to improve spoiling if the rf interpulse time is short.

The other approach for spoiling of unwanted transverse coherence is known as *rf spoiling*. Normal data acquisition techniques apply rf pulses of constant phase or with a 180° phase alternation of the excitation pulse (i.e., +90°, −90°, +90°, . . .). The receiver is also phase alternated to

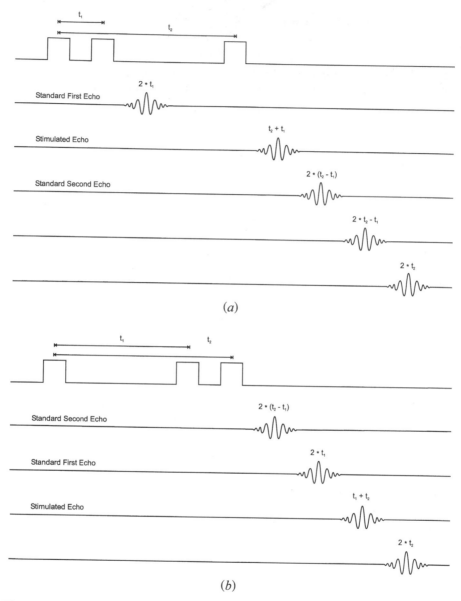

Figure 8-9. Echo timing plots. (*a*) Time t_1 is less than t_2, typical of a standard short *TE*/long *TE* spin echo pulse sequence. Five echoes are formed. Two are used in routine imaging (1 and 3). The stimulated echo occurs at time $t_1 + t_2$ (echo 2); (*b*) Time t_1 is greater than t_2, typical of a spin echo pulse sequence with a short *TE* and a spatial presaturation pulse. Four echoes are formed. Two are used in routine imaging (1 and 2). The stimulated echo occurs at time $t_1 + t_2$ (echo 3).

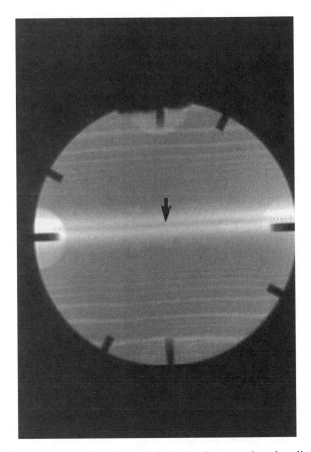

Figure 8-10. Signal contributions from undesired echoes produce banding artifacts (arrow). These echoes can be minimized through the use of coherence spoiling.

match the transmitter phase so that signal averaging can be performed. Rf spoiling applies a random phase variation to the excitation pulse and receiver. The desired echo signals add in a coherent fashion, while the other echoes add in an incoherent manner. If a sufficiently large number of phase variations is used, the net result is that the undesired signals average to zero. Rf spoiling does not require additional time during the slice loop, but does require sophisticated phase modulation of the transmitter.

8.2.6 Magnetic Susceptibility Difference Artifact

A third artifact whose appearance is sensitive to the measurement sequence is caused by differences in magnetic susceptibility χ between adjacent regions of tissue. The magnetic susceptibility is a measure of the electronic polarization induced by the external magnetic field. The degree of polarization depends on the electronic and atomic structure of the sample. Tissues such as cortical bone or air-filled organs such as lungs or bowel contain little polarizable material and have very small values for χ. Soft tissue has a greater degree of polarization and larger χ. At the interface between soft tissues and the area of different susceptibility, a significant change in the local magnetic field is present over a short distance, causing an enhanced dephasing of the protons located there. As *TE* increases, there is more time for proton dephasing to occur that causes signal loss. This dephasing is reversed by the 180° refocusing pulse in spin echo imaging since it is constant with time, but contributes to the contrast in gradient echo imaging. Magnetic susceptibility dephasing is also observed following administration of a paramagnetic contrast agent as the agent accumulates in the kidney and bladder. A significant signal loss occurs as the agent concentration in these organs increases (Figure 8-11).

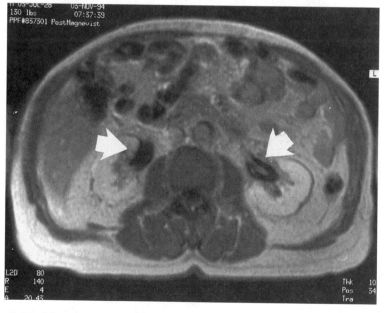

Figure 8-11. Magnetic susceptibility difference artifact. As paramagnetic contrast agents accumulate in the kidneys, the local magnetic field is distorted, causing enhanced dephasing to the protons in the vicinity and produces signal voids (arrows). Measurement parameters are: pulse sequence, spoiled gradient echo; *TR*, 140 ms; *TE*, 4 ms; acquisition matrix, 128 phase-encoding steps, 256 readout data points with twofold oversampling; *FOV*, 263 × 350 mm²; acquisition, 1.

Metal implants will have very small or very large values for χ, depending on the metal composition. In general, metal will deform the local magnetic field homogeneity surrounding it, producing significant artifacts. These artifacts frequently appear as an expansive rounded signal void with peripheral areas of high signal intensity distorting the surrounding regions, termed a "blooming" artifact. The size and shape of the artifact depends on the size, shape, orientation, and nature of the metal and the pulse sequence used for the measurement (Figure 8-12). Titanium or tantalum produce very localized distortions, while stainless steel can produce severe distortions that may compromise the images (Figure 8-13). All echoes are affected by the presence of the metal. Gradient echo sequences are much more sensitive to metal distortions. In some instances, only spin echo sequences may produce acceptable images. Fast spin echo techniques with very long echo trains are least sensitive to these distortions, and should be used when metal is known to be in the imaging field.

8.3 EXTERNAL ARTIFACTS

External artifacts are generated from sources other than patient tissue. Their appearance in the final images depends on the nature of the source and the measurement conditions. The sources may be classified into two general categories: those originating from a malfunctioning or miscalibration of the MRI hardware and those that are not. Excluded from this group are hardware problems that cause complete failure of data collection or image reconstruction. Manufacturers exert great effort to ensure that the acquired images faithfully represent the MR signals from the defined area of interest. The artifacts described here are not specific to any particular manufacturer, but can occur on any MR system.

8.3.1 Magnetic Field Distortions

One of the most common system-related problems is produced by static distortions of the main magnetic field. During system installation, manufacturers perform a field optimization procedure known as *shimming* to eliminate coarse distortions of the central magnetic field caused by metal in the immediate vicinity of the magnet. However, patients also produce field distortions due to their nonuniform shape and tissue content. These distortions can cause contrast variations within the image, particularly when fat saturation is used. In addition, common metal ob-

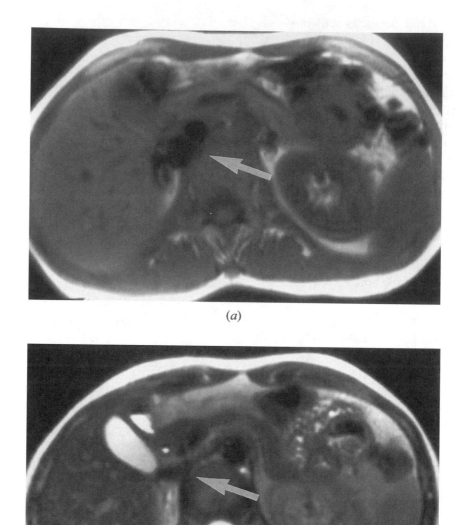

(*a*)

(*b*)

Figure 8-12. Magnetic susceptibility difference artifact. Surgical clips produce a void of signal caused due to the significant magnetic field distortion. (*a*) Spoiled gradient echo sequence shows significant signal distortion (arrow). (*b*) Single shot echo train spin echo at the same level shows minimal signal loss (arrow).

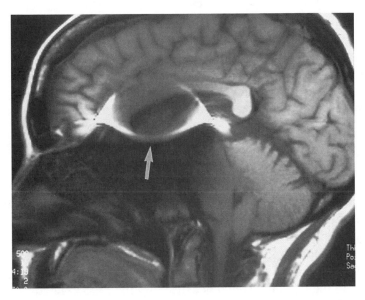

Figure 8-13. Stainless steel aneurysm clip produces severe field distortion. Pulse sequence, spin echo.

jects within the bore such as paper clips or staples can cause severe image distortion.

The amount of image distortion observed from static field inhomogeneities depends on the specific measurement technique. If the field homogeneity disruption is severe, the signal loss will be enough to preclude any image whatsoever. In general, gradient echo sequences are most sensitive to field distortions. This is due to the echo signal amplitude being a function of T2*, in which proton dephasing from magnetic field inhomogeneities is a significant factor affecting the image contrast. As in the case of magnetic susceptibility differences discussed earlier, very short *TE* values allow little time for such dephasing and result in smaller signal voids. Longer *TE* values allow more time for dephasing and can produce significant artifacts. Spin echo sequences, which include a 180° refocusing rf pulse, can also be used to minimize the intensity variations.

Another instance of magnetic field distortion occurs when fat saturation is used. As mentioned in Chapter 7, fat saturation pulses are rf pulses centered at the fat resonant frequency that saturate the fat protons, leaving only the water protons to contribute to the image. If the field homogeneity is not uniform, the fat suppression pulse may not uniformly suppress the fat and may even suppress the water within the tissue. This condition results in regions of nonuniform fat suppression within the image (see Figure 7-2*b*) and is most commonly observed at the edges of the optimized portion of the field, as can occur in images with large FOV or with extreme superior or inferior positions. It is advisable to try to center the anatomy within the magnet as much as possible and to perform field homogeneity correction with the patient inside the scanner prior to fat saturation.

8.3.2 Measurement Hardware

Hardware-induced artifacts are those produced by malfunctioning of one or more of the scanner components during the data collection. Most MR techniques perform multiple measurements on the volume of tissue, varying only a single gradient amplitude (the phase encoding gradient) from one measurement to the next. The assumption is that any amplitude variation in the detected signal is caused by the phase encoding gradient, providing the basis for localization in that direction. One of the primary requirements of the measurement hardware for this approach to succeed is that the gradient and rf transmitter systems act in a reliable and reproducible fashion. A lack of stability in the performance of either system causes modulations or distortions in the detected signal in addition to those intrinsic to the measurement. This distortion results in smearing or ghosting artifacts in the phase encoding direction throughout the entire image field. The magnitude and nature of the instability determines the amount of smearing. In many instances, the instability artifacts are indistinguishable from motion artifacts. Manufacturers perform tests during system calibration to assess the stability of the various systems to ensure that their performance is reproducible and stable.

Calibration of the measurement hardware is another important contribution to high-quality MR imaging. The gradient, rf transmitter, and receiver systems are calibrated to ensure their proper performance. Improper calibration produces variable distortions, depending on which component is considered. Nonlinear gradient pulses or improper amplitude calibration cause incorrect spatial localization and/or image distortion (Figure 8-14). Improper rf calibration causes incorrect excitation power, which may or may not be noticeable in the resulting images. The rf power deposition as measured by the SAR will also be inaccurate. Receiver miscalibration causes incorrect amplification of the echo signal, which may result in insufficient gain so that the signal does not exceed the background noise or in excessive gain, which may cause the echo signal to exceed the digitization limits of the scanner (Figure 8-15).

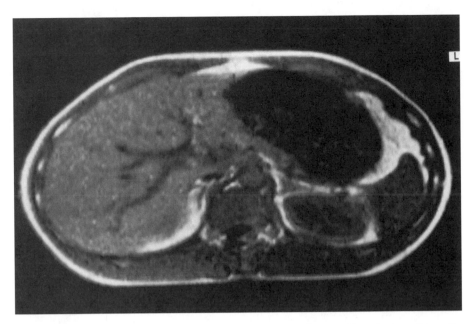

Figure 8-14. Gradient miscalibration. The phase encoding gradient is two times the correct amplitude. Note the incorrect aspect ratio.

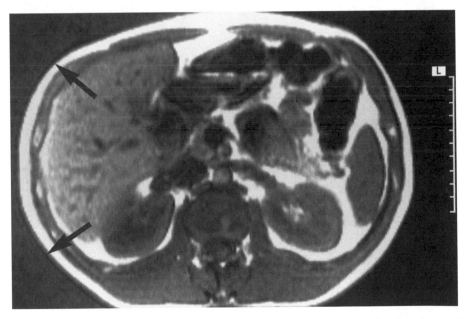

Figure 8-15. Receiver miscalibration. The measured signal is amplified in excess of the maximum input voltage for the ADC. Note the enhanced background signal (arrows).

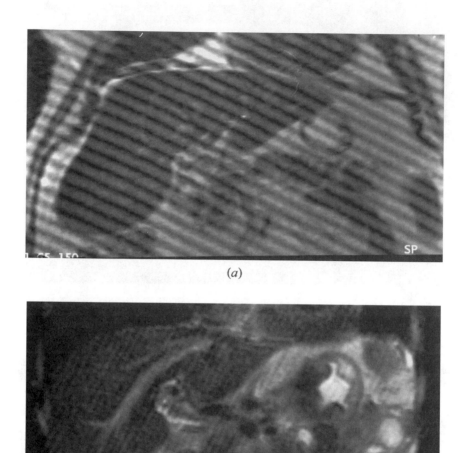

(a)

(b)

Figure 8-16. (a), (b). Spikes. Transient electrical discharges (spikes) during the data collection period produce a banding pattern that is superimposed across the entire imaging field. The direction and spacing of the bands depends on the timing of the discharge relative to the collection of the central phase encoding steps.

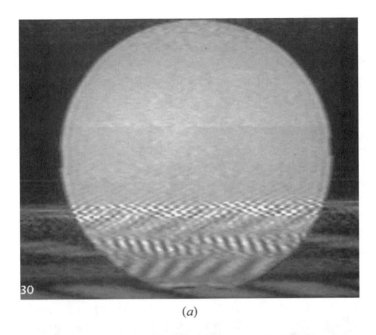

(a)

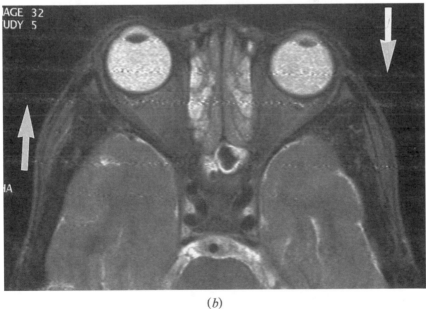

(b)

Figure 8-17. External interference. (a). Artifact due to electrical source outside the scan room. Repeated scan with scan door closed was free of artifact. (b) Interference from portable patient medication unit operating in scan room during the measurement (arrows).

8.3.3 Noise

A final artifact often present in MR images is noise. Noise can have a variety of appearances, depending on the origin and nature of the source. It may appear as a film superimposed over the normal anatomy, with or without discernible patterns, or it may have a discrete pattern or patterns. The two most common examples of noise are spikes and those arising from external sources.

Spikes are noise bursts of short duration that occur randomly during the data collection. They are normally caused by static electricity discharges or arcing of electrical components, but may be generated by many different sources. Their appearance in an image depends on the severity, number, and location of the spike in relation to the signal maximum but tend to appear as waves superimposed on the normal image data (Figure 8-16). They may or may not occur in all images of the scan. Spikes are particularly problematic to isolate because they are often irreproducible, particularly if the source is static discharge.

External interference artifacts occur when there is a source of time-varying signal detected by the receiver. They appear as lines of constant frequency within the image. Their positions depend on the receiver bandwidth of the sequence and the frequency difference from the transmitter. The most common example of this is from the alternating nature (AC) of standard electrical current (60 Hz in the United States, 50 Hz in Europe and Asia) (Figure 8-17). Electrical connections for any equipment such as external patient monitoring devices used in the scanner room are filtered before penetrating the Faraday shield or use nonalternating (DC) current. Manufacturers should be consulted before incorporating any electrical equipment into the scan room.

CHAPTER 9

Motion Artifact Reduction Techniques

As discussed in Chapter 8, motion in an MR image can produce severe image artifacts in the phase encoding direction. The severity of the artifact depends on the nature of the motion, the time during data collection when the motion occurs, and the particular pulse sequence and measurement parameters. The most critical portion of the data collection period for artifact generation is during the collection of echoes following low amplitude phase encoding steps (center of k space). Motion during the high amplitude phase encoding steps causes blurring but not severe signal misregistration in the image. Three methods are commonly used to reduce the severity of the motion artifact on the final image. Two of these, acquisition parameter modification and physiological triggering, affect the mechanics of the data collection process, while the third method, gradient motion rephasing, alters the intrinsic signal from the moving tissue. Although none of these approaches completely removes motion artifacts from the image, use of one or more of these techniques substantially reduces the impact of motion on the final images.

9.1 ACQUISITION PARAMETER MODIFICATION

Proper choice of the acquisition parameters can alter the appearance of motion artifacts. One example of this is to define the phase encoding direction so that the motion artifact does not obscure the area of interest. This may be referred to as *motion artifact rotation* or swapping the frequency and phase encoding directions. This approach does not eliminate or minimize the artifact, but only changes its position within the image. For example, motion artifacts due to eye movement or blood flow from the sagittal sinus vein may obscure lesions in the cerebrum if the phase encoding direction for a transverse slice is in the anterior-posterior direction. If the phase encoding direction is in the left-right direction, the eye motion artifacts are superimposed and lie outside the brain. The blood flow artifact also appears in an area outside the brain (Figure 9-1).

Another example of parameter modification is to increase the number of acquisitions. This approach is of particular benefit in abdominal imaging where respiratory motion can produce severe ghosting. With multiple acquisitions, the signal from the tissue is based on its average position throughout the scan. Since the tissue is in the same location most of the time, the signals add coherently. The motion artifact signal will be reduced in amplitude relative to the tissue signal.

Alternately, removal of respiratory artifacts in abdominal imaging can be accomplished by measuring all the scan data within one breath-hold. For example, a $TR = 140$ ms, $N_{PE} = 128$ and $N_{AQ} = 1$ produces a complete scan in 18 seconds. The spatial resolution may be compromised in the phase encoding direction, depending on the FOV, but respiratory motion and its artifacts will not be present if the patient suspends respiration. Extreme examples of this approach are single shot echo train spin echo and EPI techniques, where images can be acquired in less than one second producing heart and bowel images that are virtually motion-artifact free (Figure 9-2).

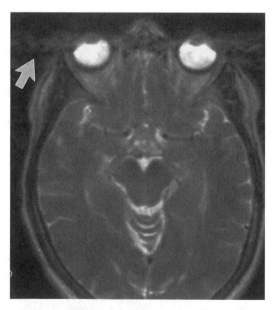

Figure 9-1. The direction of motion artifacts is determined by the phase encoding gradient. Eye movement during the scan produces motion artifact (arrow). Phase encoding: Left/Right. Readout: Anterior/Posterior.

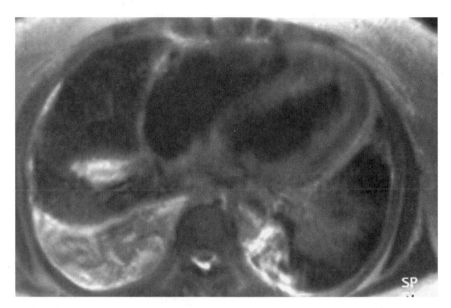

Figure 9-2. Single shot echo train spin echo image of heart acquired without triggering.

9.2 TRIGGERING/GATING

Another method of data collection that reduces motion artifacts is known as prospective triggering or gating. In this approach, the measurement is initiated following a periodic signal produced by the patient such as a pulse or heartbeat. The signal detection for a particular slice always occurs at the same time following the timing signal. Since the moving tissue is in the same relative position at this time, there is minimal misregistration of signal and a significant reduction of the resulting motion artifact. An important application of this technique is heart imaging, where data collection is synchronized to the ECG signal of the patient. The peak R wave is normally used as the timing reference point. Each phase encoding step is acquired at the same point in time following the R wave so that the heart is in the same relative position (Figure 9-3). Since the time per slice is shorter than the duration of the R–R interval, many images can be acquired within one heart beat. Two approaches are commonly used to subdivide the images. For spin echo imaging, each image is acquired at a different slice position and a different time point in the cardiac cycle. These images are typically T1 weighted (depending on the R–R time interval) with minimal blood signal, and are used for morphological studies of the heart (Figure 9-4). Another approach has significant blood signal and is known as cine heart imaging.

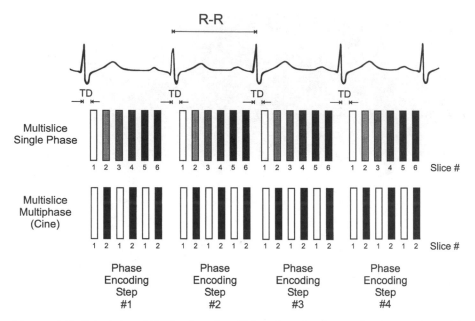

Figure 9-3. Principle of ECG triggering. Triggering the data collection to the ECG signal from the patient decreases the severity of the motion artifact. The R wave is used as an initiation signal. For multislice, single phase imaging, one phase encoding step for each slice is acquired per heartbeat. Information for a particular slice is acquired at the same time following the R wave. The T1 contrast is based on the R–R time interval rather than the user-defined *TR*. Alternately, a multislice, multiphase acquisition may be performed in which slices acquired at different times during the cardiac cycle at the same position. A trigger delay (TD) can be used to initiate data collection at any desired time during the cardiac cycle.

In this method, multiple images are acquired at each slice position during the R–R time interval. Rapid display of these images allows a dynamic visualization of the heart during the different phases of the cardiac cycle.

There are several potential problems with triggered studies. One is that the scan time is longer for a triggered study than for the corresponding untriggered study. Time must be allowed from the end of data collection to the next trigger signal to ensure that the trigger signal is properly detected by the measurement hardware. This extra time is usually 150–200 ms to allow for variation of the heart rate of the patient. The total scan time will be extended by approximately 1–2 minutes. Another problem with heart imaging occurs if the heart rate is irregular. The effective *TR* for a phase encoding step depends on the R–R time interval. Variation in the heart rate causes variation in the amount of T1 relaxation from measurement to measurement for each phase encoding

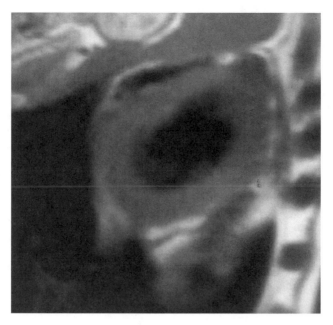

Figure 9-4. Short-axis $T1$-weighted image acquired using a triggered multislice mode.

step. This variation produces amplitude changes in the detected signal, producing misregistration artifacts in the final images even if the triggering is perfect. Stability of the heart rate is most critical during collection of the echoes following low amplitude phase encoding gradients. Finally, proper detection of the ECG signal from the patient is critical. Improper electrode placement may detect significant signal from the blood during its flow through the aortic arch. In addition, the transmitted rf energy and the gradient pulses may also interact with the lead wires, inducing significant noise to the detected ECG signal. High resistance lead wires may even burn the patient through this coupling.

An alternative to prospective triggering for cine heart imaging is known as *retrospective gating*. In this approach, the ECG signal is measured but the data collection is not controlled by the timing signal. Instead, the data are measured in an untriggered fashion and the time following the R wave when each phase encoding step was measured is stored with it. Following completion of the data collection, images are reconstructed corresponding to various time points within the cardiac cycle. The data for any phase encoding step not directly measured are interpolated from the measured values.

Gating of the measurement can also be used for abdominal imaging to reduce artifacts from respiratory motion. Two approaches are used, both of which synchronize the data collection to the respiratory cycle of the patient. A pressure transducer is positioned on the abdomen or chest to monitor the respiratory motion and produce a timing reference. Simple respiratory gating acquires the data when there is minimal motion. It suffers from significantly longer scan times since the time during respiratory motion is not used for data collection. An alternative method for T1-weighted imaging, respiratory compensation, rearranges the phase encoding gradient table so that adjacent G_{PE} are acquired when the abdomen is in the same relative position. Typically the low amplitude G_{PE} are acquired at or near end expiration so that the echoes contributing the most signal are measured when there is the least motion. Higher amplitude G_{PE} are acquired during inspiration. Significant improvement of respiratory-induced ghosts can be achieved by either technique as long as there is a uniform respiration rate during the scan. Nonuniform respiration may produce artifacts as severe as those produced from a nongated scan.

9.3   GRADIENT MOTION REPHASING

A final method for reducing motion artifacts uses additional gradient pulses to correct for phase shifts experienced by the moving protons. It is known as *gradient motion rephasing* (GMR), *motion artifact suppression technique* (MAST), or *flow compensation*. As described in Chapter 5, a gradient echo is generated by the application of two gradient pulses of equal duration and magnitude but opposite polarity. Proper dephasing and rephasing of the protons and correct frequency mapping occur as long as there is no motion during the gradient pulses. Movement during either gradient pulse results in incomplete phase cancellation or a net phase accumulation at the end of the second gradient pulse time. The amount of phase accumulation is related to the velocity of the motion. This phase accumulation produces signal intensity variations that are manifest as motion artifacts in the phase encoding direction (Figure 9-5a).

If the motion of the protons is relatively simple with respect to time, then it may be analyzed mathematically using a limited Taylor series expansion. The induced phase changes can be predicted and may be corrected by applying additional gradient pulses. These pulses will be applied in the direction for which compensation is desired. The number, duration, amplitude, and timing of the pulses can be defined so that protons with constant velocity (first-order motion), acceleration (second-

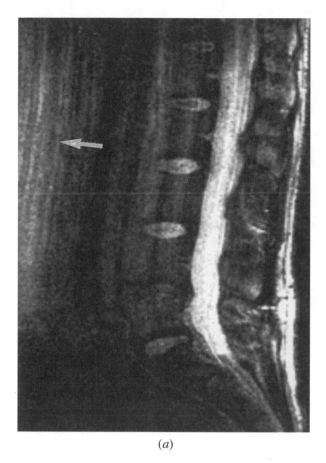

(*a*)

Figure 9-5. Gradient motion rephasing. Use of gradient motion rephasing pulses will map moving protons such as cerebrospinal fluid to their proper location. Measurement parameters are: pulse sequence, spin echo; *TR*, 2500 ms; *TE*, 90 ms; excitation angle, 90°; acquisition matrix, 192 phase-encoding steps, 256 readout data points with twofold readout oversampling; *FOV*, 210 mm PE × 280 mm RO; acquisitions, 1; slice thickness, 5 mm. (*a*) No GMR. Misregistration artifact from CSF flow appears anterior to the spinal canal (arrow). (*b*) First order GMR in readout and slice selection directions. CSF is properly mapped into the spinal canal. *Illustration continued on following page.*

order motion), and pulsatility (third-order motion) can be properly mapped within the image (Pipe). For gradient echo sequences, first-order compensation is normally sufficient for proper registration of cerebral spinal fluid, while for spin echo sequences, higher order compensation can often be achieved with minimal complications (Figure 9-5*b*).

Gradient motion rephasing requires that certain limitations be placed on the pulse sequence. Since additional gradient pulses are applied dur-

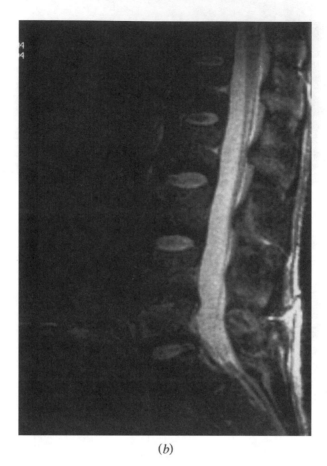

(*b*)

Figure 9-5. (*Continued*)

ing the slice loop, the minimum *TE* for the sequence must be extended to allow time for their application. In pulse sequences where short *TE*s are desired, higher amplitude gradient pulses of shorter duration may be used. This will limit the minimum *FOV* available for the sequence. In practice, only modest increases in *TE* and the minimum *FOV* are normally required.

CHAPTER 10

Magnetic Resonance Angiography

One of the main reasons that MRI has become a major technique for patient imaging is its ability to acquire information regarding the functional nature of tissue. The most common example is the examination of flowing blood within the vascular network using MR angiography (MRA). While moving tissue normally produces severe artifacts in an image, MRA uses flowing tissue as the primary source of signal intensity in the image. It provides visualization of the normal, laminar flow of blood within the vascular system and its disruptions due to pathologic conditions such as stenoses. MRA can be of particular benefit in evaluating vessel patency. MRA techniques have the advantage over conventional X-ray-based angiographic techniques in that use of a contrast agent is not always required. Consequently, multiple scans may be performed if desired (e.g., visualizing arterial then venous flow).

The most common MRA approach is a so-called bright-blood method. Signal from the moving protons is accentuated relative to the stationary protons through the pulse sequence and measurement parameters. Bright-blood MRA techniques can be divided into two approaches: time-of-flight and phase contrast methods. Both methods visualize arterial and venous flow simultaneously through the volume of interest in their simplest implementation, which can lead to ambiguous identification if the vessels are in close proximity to each other. One way to select either arterial or venous flow is to apply spatial presaturation pulses to saturate the undesired blood signal prior to its entry into the imaging volume (Figure 10-1). Presaturation pulses may also be used in "black blood" techniques where the blood signal is saturated and the vessels appear dark relative to the surrounding tissue.

MRA techniques use gradient echo sequences as the measurement technique and may use 2D-sequential or 3D-volume acquisition modes. Gradient echo sequences allow the use of short *TE* times (usually less than 10 msec), which minimize T2* dephasing of the blood signal. The choice of 2D versus 3D is usually dictated based on the total volume of tissue to be examined and by the total measurement time. 3D techniques

129

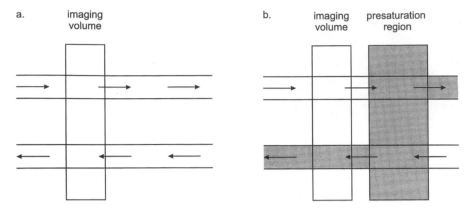

Figure 10-1. Flow selection in MR angiography. (*a*) In the absence of presaturation pulse, flowing blood entering the imaging volume is visualized regardless of the direction of the flow. (*b*) A presaturation pulse that saturates flowing blood prior to its entry into the imaging volume suppresses signal from that volume.

provide the best in-plane resolution and minimize vessel misregistration. However, saturation of blood at the distal side of the volume limits the slab thickness to approximately 70 mm unless a T1 relaxation agent is used. 3D methods require significantly longer scan times. The 2D-sequential mode is preferable for imaging vessels of slow flow such as veins or to limit saturation effects from in-plane flow. Coverage of large areas of anatomy is possible in one measurement since the volume of excitation is typically 3–4 mm per slice.

There are two additional problems associated with MRA. One is that the saturation pulse becomes less effective as more time elapses between the presaturation and the excitation pulse. This problem occurs both due to increased T1 relaxation of the blood as well as time-of-flight effects (see Section 10.1). It can be minimized by proper positioning of the presaturation pulse near the volume of excitation. A second problem is an exaggerated sensitivity to vessel stenosis. The stenotic region disrupts the laminar flow in the area of and distal to the stenosis, causing a loss of signal from the vessel greater than from the stenotic region alone. As the laminar flow is reestablished within the vessel, bright signal can again be measured.

10.1 TIME-OF-FLIGHT MRA

Time-of-flight techniques are the most time-efficient methods for obtaining MRA images. A single measurement is performed, with the stationary tissue signal suppressed relative to the flowing tissue signal. A *TR* much shorter than the tissue T1 values and a moderate excitation angle are used to accomplish this. While the stationary tissue experiences every rf excitation pulse, the flowing tissue does not. A volume of blood will be at a different location at the time of each excitation pulse due to its motion during *TR* (Figure 10-2). The signal from the blood volume is largest at the entry point of the slice because it has not undergone any excitation pulses. As the blood volume travels through the slice, it becomes saturated as it undergoes more excitation pulses and loses signal. If the flow direction is perpendicular to the slice (through-plane flow), and the volume of excitation is small, then the volume of blood exits the slice before it is completely saturated and significant blood signal can be measured throughout the entire slice. The degree of blood saturation depends on the slice thickness, *TR*, excitation angle, and flow velocity.

Time-of-flight techniques suffer from incomplete suppression of the stationary tissue due to the faster T1 relaxation times of the stationary tissues relative to the blood. Magnetization transfer (MT) pulses are often incorporated for additional suppression of the stationary tissue to enhance the ability for small vessel detection (Figure 10-3). Three-

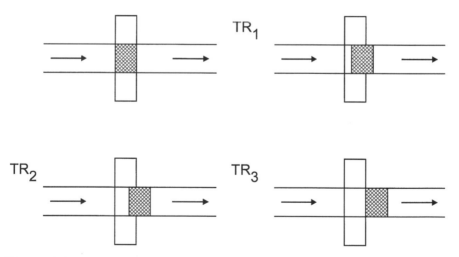

Figure 10-2. Time-of-flight effect. During data collection, the imaging volume experiences many rf pulses. Flowing blood (hashed box) experiences the first rf pulse (upper left). During the first *TR* period, the excited blood moves (upper right) and only a portion experiences the second rf pulse. During the second *TR* time period, the initial volume of blood continues to move (lower left). By the end of a third *TR* time period, the initial volume of blood is entirely outside the volume of excitation and does not contribute to the detected signal (lower right).

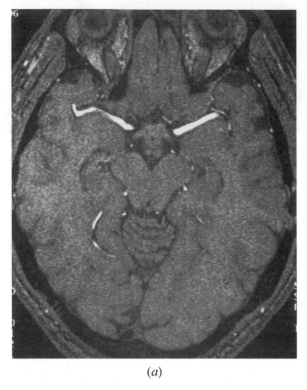

(*a*)

Figure 10-3. Time-of-flight MRA showing effects of magnetization transfer pulse. Other measurement parameters are: pulse sequence, 3D refocused gradient echo, post-excitation; *TR*, 35 ms; *TE*, 7 ms; excitation angle, 25°; acquisition matrix, 192 phase-encoding steps, 512 readout data points with twofold readout oversampling; *FOV*, 201 mm PE × 230 mm RO; acquisitions, 1; effective slice thickness, 0.78 mm. (*a*) Source image without MT pulse; (*b*) Transverse postprocessed image of Figure 10-3*a*; (*c*) Source image, one from data set acquired with MT pulse; (*d*) Transverse postprocessed image of Figure 10-3*c*. Note reduction of background gray and white matter in (*c*) compared to (*a*) (arrow) and improved visualization of vessels in (*d*) compared to (*b*) (arrow).

dimensional time-of-flight techniques also have increased saturation of the blood due to the large number of excitation pulses. For this reason, they are suitable only for vessels with fast flow such as moderate-sized arteries. Two approaches have been developed to overcome this saturation. In one method, the excitation pulse is modified to produce a ramped or nonuniform range of excitation angles across the imaging volume (Figure 10-4). Increased excitation energy is applied to protons at the distal side of the imaging volume. This induces more transverse magnetization and more signal from the more saturated protons (Figure

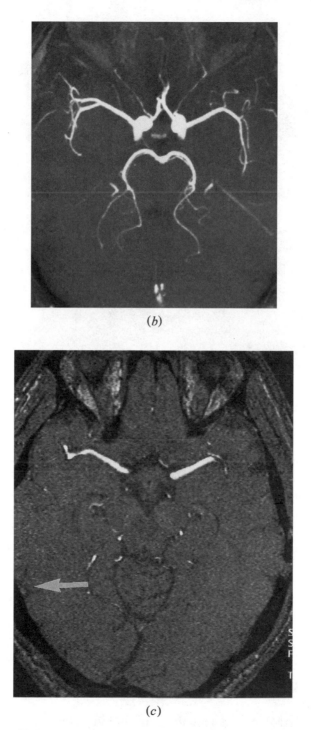

(b)

(c)

Figure 10-3. (*Continued*) *Illustration continued on following page.*

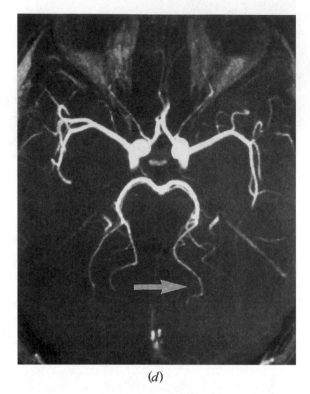

(*d*)

Figure 10-3. (*Continued*)

10-5). A second approach to obtain more blood signal uses T1 contrast agents to shorten the T1 relaxation time of blood. This approach is particularly useful for visualization of abdominal arteries using 3D time-of-flight techniques (Figure 10-6). Measurement times can be reduced to a few seconds, enabling suspension of respiration during the scan. Use of contrast agents for abdominal MRA has enabled rapid, reliable, and high-quality studies to be obtained with minimal contamination from patient motion. Studies of peripheral vessels by MRA can also be performed following contrast administration. Multilevel acquisitions together with rapid movement of the patient table allows for run-off studies of extremities within a single short imaging session.

10.2 PHASE CONTRAST MRA

Phase contrast MRA is a technique in which background tissue signal is subtracted from the flow-enhanced image to produce flow-only im-

a.   b.

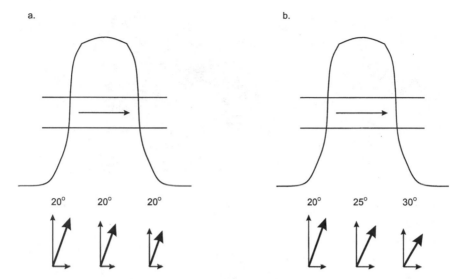

Figure 10-4. TONE rf pulse. (*a*) Normal excitation pulses provide uniform energy deposition across the slice, which gradually increases saturation of and reduces the transverse magnetization from blood located at the exit side of the slice, causing a loss of signal. (*b*) Nonuniform excitation pulses known as *ramped* or tilted optimized non-uniform excitation (*TONE*) *rf pulses* increase the excitation across the slice. While the amount of saturation increases, the resulting transverse magnetization remains constant so that the blood signal remains uniform throughout the imaging volume.

ages, analogous to digital subtraction X-ray angiography. The acquisition sequence may produce a one-dimensional profile, or standard 2D or 3D images. A minimum of two images is measured at each slice position. One image, known as the reference image, is acquired with gradient motion rephasing (see Chapter 9). Subsequent images are acquired following application of additional gradient pulses that induce a phase shift in blood moving with a particular flow velocity and direction. The selected protons are rephased at the echo time *TE* and subtracted from the reference image to produce images of only the moving protons. Additional scans may be performed to sensitize flow in other directions. The resultant difference images may be combined to produce images sensitive to flow in any direction at the chosen velocity.

Phase contrast MRA has several advantages over time-of-flight techniques. Being subtraction rather than saturation techniques, they have better background suppression than time-of-flight methods. Through their directional sensitization, phase contrast methods enable flow in each primary direction to be separately visualized. In addition, quantitation of the flow velocity in each direction is possible. However, phase

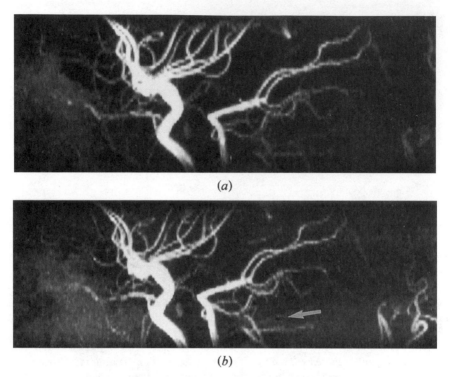

(a)

(b)

Figure 10-5. Time-of-flight MRA showing effects of TONE rf pulse. Other measurement parameters are: pulse sequence, 3D refocused gradient echo, postexcitation; *TR*, 35 ms; *TE*, 7 ms; excitation angle, 25°; acquisition matrix, 192 phase-encoding steps, 512 readout data points with twofold readout oversampling; *FOV*, 201 × 230 mm²; acquisitions, 1; effective slice thickness, 0.78 mm. (*a*) Sagittal projection of volume using normal uniform excitation pulse; (*b*) Sagittal projection of volume using TONE excitation pulse. Note improved signal from vessels (arrow).

contrast methods suffer from two problems. One is a significantly longer scan time. Four separate acquisitions are required to measure all three flow components. The scan time is four times longer than for a time-of-flight method with similar acquisition parameters. In addition, prior knowledge of the maximum velocity is necessary to ensure that the

Figure 10-6. MR angiography of aorta and renal arteries following bolus administration of gadolinium-chelate contrast agent. Measurement parameters are: pulse sequence, 3D refocused gradient echo, postexcitation; *TR*, 15 ms; *TE*, 2 ms; excitation angle, 15°; acquisition matrix, 128 phase-encoding steps, 256 readout data points with twofold readout oversampling; *FOV*, 400 × 400 mm²; acquisitions, 1; effective slice thickness, 2.0 mm. (*a*) Source image, one from data set. (*b*) Coronal postprocessed image.

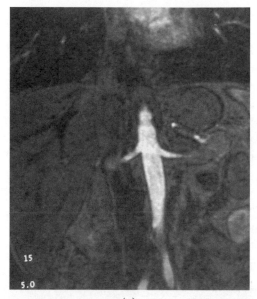

(a)

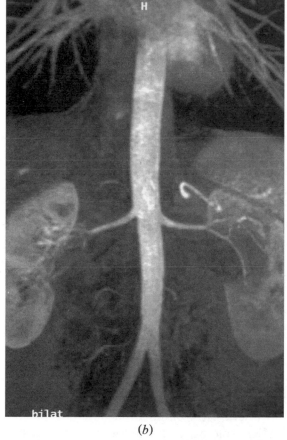

(b)

137

proper sensitization pulse is used. The maximum signal is achieved for blood flowing at the sensitive velocity. Flow velocities exceeding this velocity are misregistered as slower flow, a situation known as *aliasing*. This artifact is analogous to the high frequency aliasing problem observed in phase encoding (see Chapter 4). Blood signal is reduced at these higher velocities until a complete loss of flow signal occurs at flow velocities that are multiples of the sensitive velocity. At the other extreme, a sensitive velocity too large will minimize contrast between velocity changes within a vessel. Proper choice of the sensitive velocity allows adequate visualization of all flow with good sensitivity to velocity variations within a vessel.

10.3   MAXIMUM INTENSITY PROJECTION

Regardless of the choice of acquisition technique, examination of the individual images from an MRA scan can provide details regarding flow variations within a vessel. However, a vessel is seldom located within a single slice but usually extends through several slices at an arbitrary angle, making vessel tortuosity and the spatial relationship with neighboring vessels difficult to assess, particularly if the vessels are oriented perpendicular to the imaging volume. Bright-blood MRA images may be analyzed using a postprocessing technique known as *maximum intensity projection* (MIP) to better visualize the three-dimensional vessel topography.

The MIP process generates images from the entire set of MRA images. A view direction is chosen and the entire set of images is projected along that direction onto a perpendicular plane using a "ray tracing" approach. The pixel of maximum intensity is chosen as the pixel for the MIP image, regardless of the input slice where the pixel is located (Figure 10-7). Because the bright-blood MRA technique accentuates blood signal over stationary tissue signal, the MIP process preferentially selects blood vessels whenever possible, which enables the entire vessel to be examined no matter where it is located within the imaging volume. Multiple images may be obtained from the same data set through change of the view direction (rotation of the projection angle). Vessels that may be superimposed in one projection can be clearly resolved in another one. It is also possible to perform the MIP process on a subset of the data, a so-called targeted approach. This is useful for isolating the left and right carotid arteries, for elimination of suborbital or subcutaneous fat in cerebral MRA studies, or for tailored reconstruction of the renal

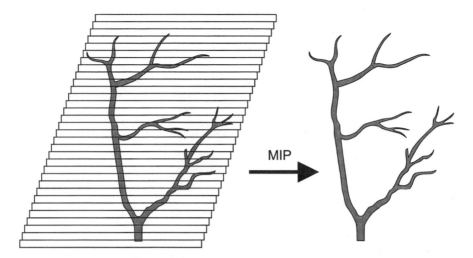

Figure 10-7. Maximum intensity projection (MIP). The MR images are acquired so that moving blood has pixels of maximal intensity. The MIP process maps the pixels of maximum intensity into a single projection or view regardless of which slice the pixel was located in. Changing the direction of projection provides a different perspective of the vessels.

arteries. Care must be taken in the definition of the targeted area that the vessel of interest does not leave the area. The MIP process causes the vessel to be cut off at the edge of the defined region, simulating a vessel obstruction. Careful examination of the source images is necessary to ensure the inclusion of the entire vessel within the reconstructed area.

CHAPTER 11

Advanced Imaging Applications

Initially, MR imaging was restricted to visualizing hydrogen nuclei using basic spin echo techniques. As hardware and software have evolved, newer and faster imaging techniques have been developed. The advent of subsecond imaging techniques has provided the ability to measure metabolic processes within tissues with significantly faster temporal resolution than was previously possible. Also, imaging of nuclei other than hydrogen has become more feasible. Four such applications are described in this chapter: diffusion, perfusion, functional imaging, and imaging of hyperpolarized noble gases.

11.1 DIFFUSION

As mentioned in Chapter 1, all matter is made of atoms, which bond to form molecules. These molecules continually move due to interactions with their surroundings. Two types of movement are found in tissues. One is coherent bulk flow, which occurs for blood or cerebrospinal fluid. This movement arises from a difference in pressure between the two locations, produced by contractions of the heart. Direct visualization of blood flow within the vascular network is accomplished using MR angiographic techniques, as described in Chapter 10.

Another manifestation of this continuous movement of molecules is a relatively small displacement of the molecule in space, known as *translational motion*. Although many processes in nature can cause translational motion, one of the most important ones in biological systems is diffusion. Diffusion of molecules occurs due to a concentration difference between two environments, such as on either side of a cell membrane. Diffusion is thermodynamic in origin and is a nonequilibrium process responsible for the random transport of gases and nutrients from the extracellular space into the cell interior. The transit occurs from a region of high concentration to low concentration, analogous to heat flow between hot and cold regions. Diffusion is characterized by a constant known as the *diffusion coefficient D*, which describes the amount of material transported across the membrane.

In biological systems, measurements of diffusion in tissue are complicated by perfusional blood flow (see Section 11.2). Blood flow through randomly oriented microscopic blood vessels results in a loss of signal, known as intravoxel incoherent motion, that is indistinguishable from diffusion. For this reason, measurements of diffusion in tissues in vivo measure a constant referred to as the *apparent diffusion coefficient* (ADC).

Studies of diffusion have been performed using MR for many years. The standard method uses a symmetric pair of gradient pulses to increase the amount of proton dephasing observed in a spin echo (Figure 11-1). Known as the Stejskal-Tanner method (Stejskal and Tanner, 1963), protons that move during the pulses experience unequal effects from the gradient pulses and do not rephase at the echo time *TE*. This causes a loss in signal amplitude from those protons:

$$S(TE) \propto \exp(-TE/T2) * \exp(-bD') \qquad [11\text{-}1]$$

where D' is the apparent diffusion coefficient, T, t, and G are defined in Figure 11-1 and

$$b = \gamma^2 G^2 t^2 (T - t/3) \qquad [11\text{-}2]$$

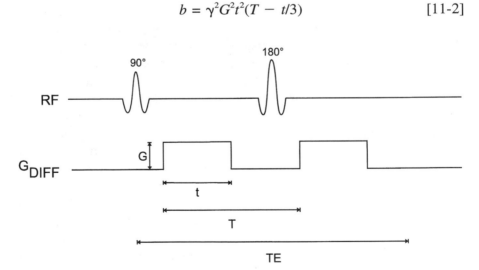

Figure 11-1. Spin echo pulse sequence showing diffusion gradients, known as the Stejskal-Tanner approach. G is the amplitude for each of the gradient pulses, t is the duration of the gradient pulse during which the diffusion weighting occurs, and T is the time between the two pulses.

The sensitivity to motion for the technique is determined by the "b" value. Larger b values can be obtained through larger gradient amplitudes, longer duration gradient pulses, or longer times between the gradient pulses. MRI applications of this technique are referred to as *diffusion-weighted imaging*. Tissues with small ADCs undergo little motion and sustain little signal loss in the image. Tissues with large ADCs move significantly during the gradient pulses and produce a significantly attenuated signal.

One of the most important applications of diffusion-weighted imaging is in the evaluation of cerebral ischemia and stroke. Normal cells maintain a concentration gradient of sodium ions extracellular and potassium ions intracellular, and are surrounded by and contain water. This enzymatic process, known as *active transport* or the *sodium-potassium-ATP pump*, requires oxygen for the production of adenosine triphosphate (ATP). The oxygen for this process is carried to the tissue from the lungs bound to hemoglobin in erythrocytes. Following the onset of ischemia and the loss of oxygen by the tissue, the ADC of the affected tissue water has been observed to decrease, leading to a decrease in dephasing and an increase in signal amplitude (Figure 11-2). Although the reason for this decrease in ADC is unclear, it is presumably due to a change in the membrane permeability to the sodium and potassium ions and an accompanying increase in intracellular water content. This ADC decrease is reversible upon restoration of blood flow, provided it occurs before complete cell membrane breakdown.

11.2   PERFUSION

Although angiographic techniques visualize the vascular network within a patient, they do not have sufficient spatial resolution to visualize blood flow through a tissue in bulk. However, it is possible in many instances to observe changes in tissue signal due to the blood flow through it, a process known as *perfusion*. Proper tissue perfusion is critical to ensure an adequate supply of nutrients to the constituent cells as well as removal of metabolic byproducts. It also aids in maintenance of a stable tissue temperature. Abnormalities in perfusion can lead to an increased temperature sensitivity and a loss of tissue viability through hypoxia.

Two approaches are used for MR perfusion studies, both of which are based on radioisotope tracer studies and use similar methods for analysis of the flow dynamics. One approach acquires a series of rapid (less than 20 seconds per image) T1-weighted imaging studies following

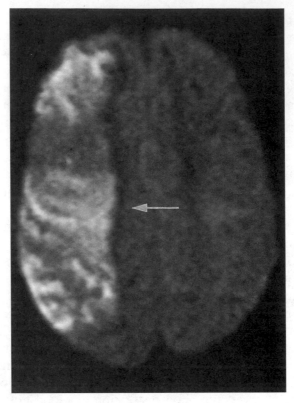

Figure 11-2. Diffusion-weighted EPI sequence. Normal tissue has moderate diffusion of water, while tissue under stress, such as that at risk for a stroke, has restricted motion of tissue water and shows increased signal (arrow).

the bolus administration of a contrast agent. These are typically acquired using spoiled gradient echo, T1-weighted magnetization prepared, or echo planar techniques. An increase in tissue signal occurs as the contrast agent infiltrates the tissue. This approach is successful if the contrast agent enters the intravascular spaces of the tissue. Perfusion defects are visualized as a lack of signal increase for the affected region of tissue. The other approach is useful if the contrast agent remains in the blood vessels, such as in cerebral tissue with an intact blood brain barrier. In this case, the paramagnetic nature of the contrast agent increases the local tissue susceptibility, causing increased T2* dephasing of nearby tissues. Serial T2*-weighted gradient echo sequences are acquired, and the well-perfused tissue has a reduction of signal relative to the precontrast images or the poorly perfused tissues.

Two examples where perfusion studies have shown promise are in the examination of abnormalities of blood flow within tissue and for the detection of tumors. Blood flow anomalies in the myocardium following infarction have been studied for many years using radionuclide agents. First-pass MR perfusion studies have shown good correlation with these studies and have enabled visualization of different phases of perfusion (Edelman and Li, 1994). Liver studies following administration of gadolinium-chelate contrast agents have also demonstrated differences in tissue perfusion. Images acquired immediately following contrast administration show capillary phase perfusion, whereas images acquired 45 seconds postadministration show substantial portal phase perfusion (Figure 11-3). The normal spleen usually shows a serpigenous enhancement pattern immediately following contrast administration, with a more uniform signal intensity observed on images acquired 45 seconds or later.

The other studies where differential perfusion has been used are in the detection of tumors. Pituitary adenomas have demonstrated a perfusional difference in microadenomas and macroadenomas following contrast administration (Finelli and Kaufman, 1993). Also, malignant breast tumors have demonstrated a significantly faster uptake of contrast media than benign tumors in some studies (Hulka et al., 1995). Rapid scanning is necessary because both classes of tumors have similar signal amplitudes 3 minutes following contrast administration. Use of a 3D volume scan enables a bilateral breast study with good spatial and temporal resolution (Figure 11-4).

11.3   FUNCTIONAL BRAIN IMAGING

An active area of research in which perfusion techniques are used is in the study of brain activity as a result of an external stimulus. The basic measurement technique is very similar to that mentioned earlier for bolus contrast agent studies of brain tissue, namely using T2*-weighted gradient echo or echo planar images. However, instead of administering an exogenous agent to reduce the T2* relaxation time, the local tissue susceptibility is shortened by the presence of endogenous paramagnetic species present in blood. As mentioned earlier in the description of diffusion-weighted imaging in the evaluation of stroke, oxygen is delivered to cells attached to hemoglobin. Deoxygenated hemoglobin has a significant paramagnetic moment, whereas oxygenated hemoglobin is diamagnetic, with a very small magnetic moment.

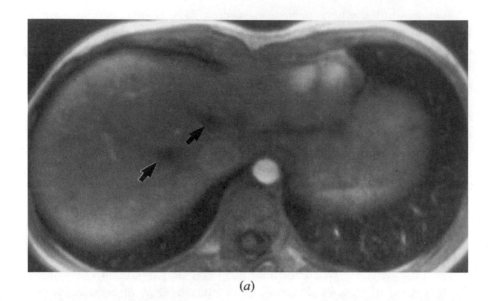

(a)

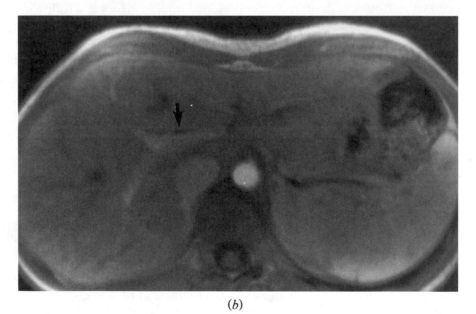

(b)

Figure 11-3. T1-weighted spoiled gradient echo imaging of liver following administration of gadolinium-chelate contrast agent. (a) Image acquired immediately following
administration. Contrast agent is in the hepatic arterial phase, as evidenced by the
nonopacified hepatic vein (arrow). (b) Image acquired 45 seconds following administration. Contrast agent is now in the capillary phase, as evidenced by its presence in
the hepatic vein (arrow).

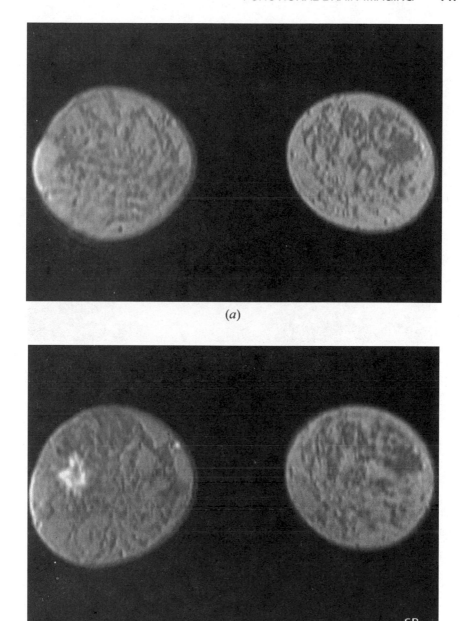

(a)

(b)

Figure 11-4. 3D-volume T1-spoiled gradient echo imaging of breast following administration of gadolinium-chelate contrast agent. (a) Precontrast image, lacking evidence of lesion. (b–d) Serial images acquired every 48 seconds following contrast agent administration. Note increased signal from lesion in later images. *Illustration continued on following page.*

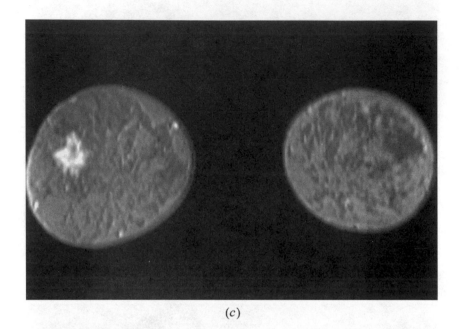

(*c*)

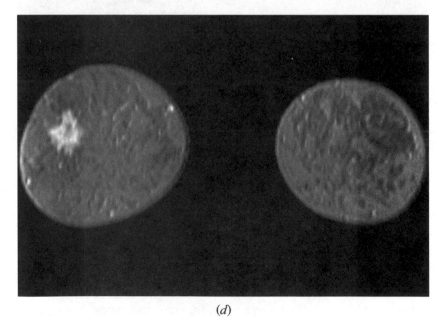

(*d*)

Figure 11-4. (*Continued*)

Brain activation studies are based on the assumption that stimulated tissue undergoes an increase in blood flow and an increased delivery of oxygenated hemoglobin. The amount of deoxygenated hemoglobin decreases within the tissue, reducing the concentration of paramagnetic species. This condition reduces the amount of susceptibility dephasing induced and thereby increases the T2* for the stimulated tissue relative to the unstimulated tissue. As a result, the stimulated tissue appears higher in signal on T2* weighted images. This process is known as the *blood oxygenation level dependent effect* or BOLD effect (DeYoe et al., 1994). The typical approach is to perform a large series of measurements in the presence and absence of the stimulus and subtract the images, leaving pixels presumably from the activated region of tissue.

The data analysis of BOLD-type functional MRI studies is an involved procedure. Correction for patient movement between the measurements must be performed. Also, the pixel intensity from the stimulated image typically exceeds that from the unstimulated image by less than 5%. This necessitates the repetition of the measurement many times (1000 or more) to ensure that the observed signal variation from the voxel is real and not artifactual in origin. The correlation coefficient of the voxel intensity and the time variation of the stimulus is also calculated to ensure that the observed variation is in response to the stimulus. A threshold of significance, known as the *z score*, must also be defined for the particular study below which the signal difference is assumed not to be relevant.

BOLD-type functional MRI studies have been used for studying many areas of the brain, including the visual, auditory, motor, and frontal cortex. Their results have compared favorably with those obtained using positron emission tomography (PET). Simple stimuli such as flashing lights or finger tapping have been used successfully. More complex stimuli such as cognitive processes are currently being evaluated.

11.4 NOBLE GAS IMAGING

As discussed in Chapter 1, the most common nucleus observed in MRI is ^{1}H, due to its high natural abundance and its large nuclear magnetic moment. In spite of these advantages, the net magnetization produced in patients by the ^{1}H atoms in water or fat through the Zeeman interaction at normal imaging magnetic fields is very small and induces a weak signal. Other attempts at measuring MR signals from endogenous nuclei such as ^{23}Na have succeeded, but their low sensitivity has limited their practical implementation.

Recently, MR imaging studies of lung air spaces using hyperpolarized ^{3}He and ^{129}Xe gases have been reported (MacFall et al., 1996; Mugler et al., 1997). Visualizing lung air spaces using normal ^{1}H imaging is difficult due to low concentration of water in air, large magnetic susceptibility differences due to the paramagnetic nature of oxygen, and artifacts from respiratory or cardiac motion. Although the latter two problems can be minimized using rapid scan techniques with short *TE* times, the low signal amplitude produced by water vapor cannot. Helium and xenon are noble gases that are relatively unreactive and dissolve into tissues readily. They can rapidly permeate into the lung spaces. They are also well tolerated by most patients, with the most common side effect being a mild sedative effect produced by xenon.

The source of the MRI signal from noble gases is spin polarization between the parallel and antiparallel orientations just as for any MR measurement, but it is produced in a different manner. Rather than use

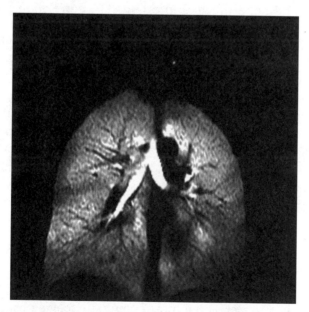

Figure 11-5. ^{3}He image of normal lung acquired following inhalation of hyperpolarized helium gas. Note significant signal in trachea and upper lobes of lungs and lack of signal from other tissue in the body. Measurement parameters are pulse sequence, 2-D refocused gradient echo, postexcitation; *TR*, 25 ms; *TE*, 10 ms; acquisition matrix, 128 phase-encoding steps, 256 readout data points; FOV, 350 × 350 mm^2. (*Image courtesy of James R. MacFall, Duke University*).

the natural spin polarization produced by the MRI magnet, these gases are polarized outside the patient through the use of a laser and rubidium atoms. The rubidium atoms are excited by the laser, and transfer the energy to the particular gas (He or Xe). This results in a net magnetization 10,000–100,000 times that produced by the MRI magnet. This hyperpolarized gas is then inhaled by the patient through a ventilator bag. Gradient echo imaging techniques are used to produce images until the net magnetization is completely lost through T2 relaxation (approximately one minute following inhalation) (Figure 11-5).

There are several technical difficulties in performing noble gas imaging. First, the ^{3}He and ^{129}Xe active isotopes are not the predominant isotopes for these atoms (see Table 1-1). For this reason, they are relatively expensive and recovery of the gas following patient studies is performed to reduce the expense. Second, the resonant frequencies for these nuclei are very different from ^{1}H so that the transmitter and receiver coils are different from those used in standard MRI studies. Third, this technique is a single-pass study. Because of the method used to produce the net magnetization, there is no possibility for a repeat measurement following inhalation. Finally, only gradient echo techniques are possible. Spin echoes require 180° refocusing pulses and the recovery of net magnetization through T1 relaxation prior to subsequent excitation pulses. There is no reformation of the net magnetization of hyperpolarized noble gases once it is dephased.

CHAPTER 12

Magnetic Resonance Spectroscopy

Although MRI is the most common application of the MR phenomenon used in the medical community, it is a relatively recent development. The original application of magnetic resonance is MR spectroscopy (MRS), a technique that allows examination of individual molecules or portions of molecules within a sample. The development of whole body scanners has allowed MRS to be used to study the biochemical nature of disease processes within a patient without the need for invasive procedures. Many of the principles of MRS are the same as those of MRI, although their focus is somewhat different. While theoretically possible on any MRI system, most MRS studies are performed using magnets of 1.5T or higher, due to the low intrinsic sensitivity of the technique. Hydrogen spectroscopic studies can be performed on standard imaging systems with no additional hardware required. This chapter summarizes some of the basic concepts of hydrogen MRS. For more complete discussions of the field see Salibi and Brown, 1998 and Mukherji, 1998.

12.1 ADDITIONAL CONCEPTS

A description of the basic principles of MRS begins at the same place as that of a description of the principles of MRI. The basic concepts of net magnetization from a collection of spins in a magnetic field, signal production following absorption of rf energy, and T1 and T2 relaxation as described in Chapters 1 through 3 are identical for MRS and MRI. However, there are two important differences between MRS and MRI. First, MRS signals are detected in the absence of a gradient. All molecules are detected in the presence of the same base magnetic field. The chemical shift described in Chapter 2 is the only source of magnetic field variation present during signal detection. Rather than be the source of artifactual signal as it is in MRI, the chemical shift is the means by which molecular species are identified in MRS studies. Second, unlike MRI, relaxation effects are avoided as much as possible in MRS studies.

The molecules under observation are relatively small in size and have relatively long T1 and T2 values. Long *TR* (typically >1500 ms) are used in order to minimize T1 saturation effects. T2 dephasing effects are dominated by main field inhomogeneities and are more properly described by T2*.

12.1.1   Spin Coupling

In addition to the chemical shift, there is another molecular interaction that modifies the environment of a proton. Protons located on the same molecule interact with each other and each has its local magnetic field affected. The most common instance of this in biological systems is facilitated by the bonding electrons in the molecule and is known as *spin coupling* or *J coupling*. Spin coupling differs from the chemical shift in two very important ways: It is independent of magnetic field strength (chemical shifts increase with B_0 when measured in Hz) and there is always another spin involved in the coupling.

Spin coupling involves a pairing interaction between spins on the same molecule that causes the MR signal of each member to be divided. The number of resultant signals and their relative amplitudes depend on the number of spins of each type. For hydrogen MRS studies in biological systems, the molecule where spin coupling is most easily viewed is lactate, $CH_3CHOHCOO^-$. Attached to the middle carbon of the molecule is a methyl group and a hydrogen atom. The hydrogen atom can be oriented parallel or antiparallel to B_0. The methyl group will sense slightly different molecular magnetic fields in each case. On average, there will be an equal number of possibilities for the hydrogen atom in each orientation, so the signal detected for the methyl group is split into two peaks separated by approximately 7 Hz, centered about the chemical shift for the methyl group. The 7 Hz value is referred to as the coupling constant *J* for this particular coupling. In a similar fashion, the methyl protons can be arranged in one of four configurations: all three parallel to B_0, all three antiparallel to B_0, two parallel and one antiparallel to B_0, or one parallel and two antiparallel to B_0. The last two configurations occur three times more frequently than the first two, so that the hydrogen atom will be divided into four peaks with relative amplitudes $1:3:3:1$ each separated by 7 Hz. Because of its low amplitude and its nearness to the water resonant frequency, this resonance is normally not visualized in vivo MRS studies.

An important feature of spin coupling is that it is not reversed by the application of a 180° refocusing rf pulse. As discussed below, one

a.   b.

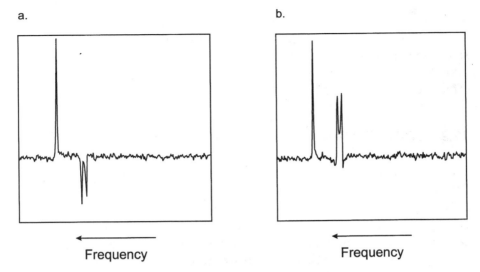

Frequency   Frequency

Figure 12-1. PRESS ^{1}H spectra of lactate (doublet) and acetate (singlet). Choice of *TE* affects the relative polarity of lactate peak compared to acetate, due to modulation of spin-coupled hydrogen atoms. Other measurement parameters are: *TR*, 1500 ms; number of acquisitions, 8; number of sample points, 1024; Volume size, 20 × 20 × 20 mm³. (*a*) *TE* = 135 ms; (*b*) *TE* = 270 ms.

method of spatial localization uses 180° refocusing rf pulses to produce a spin echo. The lactate signal is modulated in amplitude, based on the elapsed time between the rf pulses, which means that the lactate protons may or may not be in phase with the other protons at the echo time *TE*. This condition is analogous to the phase modulation seen in gradient echo MRI studies for fat and water. The rate of this modulation is proportional to 1/*J*. For the 7 Hz coupling, it corresponds to a phase modulation period of approximately 270 ms. Use of a *TE* of 270 ms ensures that the lactate resonances are in phase with the other noncoupled resonances, while use of a *TE* of 135 ms has the lactate signals 180° out of phase with the other resonances (Figure 12-1).

12.1.2 Water Suppression

Clinical MRI techniques visualize the water and fat within the desired slice. The high concentration of water and fat within the tissue makes this feasible. In MRS, the metabolites under observation are as much as 10,000 times less concentrated than water, which makes their detection in the presence of tissue water difficult. In order to accomplish this, suppression of the water is necessary. The most common approach uses a frequency selective rf pulse centered at the water resonant frequency to saturate the water protons. This technique is analogous to the fat saturation pulse described in Chapter 7. Water suppression factors of 100 or more are possible from a single pulse, making it an easy and effective way for reducing the signal contamination from water.

12.2   LOCALIZATION TECHNIQUES

Current techniques used for spatial localization of the MRS signals were derived from similar techniques used in MRI. Slice selective excitation pulses in conjunction with gradient pulses are used to localize the rf energy to the desired volume of tissue, in the same manner as described in Chapter 4. However, unlike MRI, where the voxel size is typically 5 $\times$ 1 $\times$ 1 mm^3 or less, MRS voxel sizes are usually 15 $\times$ 15 $\times$ 15 mm^3 or larger. Therefore MRS studies are limited to the examination of relatively large regions of tissue. The two general categories of localization techniques are based on the number of separate voxels from which spectra are obtained in each measurement.

12.2.1   Single Voxel Techniques

Single voxel techniques (also called *single voxel spectroscopy* or SVS) acquire spectra from a single small volume of tissue. The most common approaches excite only the desired tissue volume through the intersection of three rf excitation pulses. Two schemes of rf pulses are used. The first approach, known as *point resolved spectroscopy* (PRESS), uses a 90° and two 180° rf pulses in a fashion similar to a standard multiecho sequence (Figure 12-2). Each rf pulse is applied using a different physical gradient as the slice selection gradient. Only protons located at the intersection of all three pulses produce the spin echo at the desired *TE*. The other approach, known as *stimulated echo acquisition method* (STEAM), uses three 90° rf pulses, each with a different slice selection gradient (Figure 12-3). The resulting stimulated echo (see Section 8.2.5, Coherence Artifacts) is produced by protons located at the intersection of the pulses.

There are several differences between PRESS and STEAM. The major difference is in the nature of the echo signal. In PRESS, the entire net magnetization from the voxel is refocused to produce the echo signal, whereas in STEAM, a maximum of one-half of the entire net magnetization generates the stimulated echo. As a result, PRESS has a S/N ratio significantly larger than for STEAM. PRESS uses 180° rf pulses while

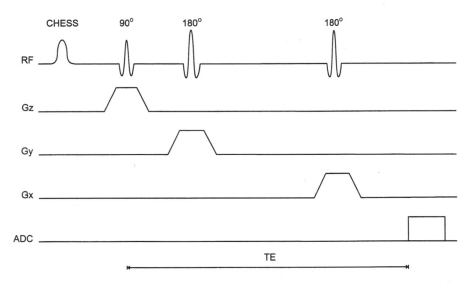

Figure 12-2. PRESS pulse sequence timing diagram. The CHESS rf pulse is used for suppression of water.

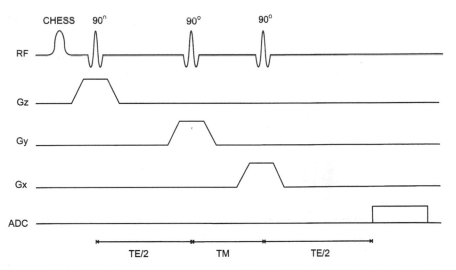

Figure 12-3. STEAM pulse sequence timing diagram. The CHESS rf pulse is used for suppression of water.

STEAM uses only 90° rf pulses. The voxel dimensions with PRESS may be limited by the high transmitter power for the 180° rf pulses. STEAM spectra are also unaffected by J coupling of spins, while PRESS spectra show a modulation of the signal from any coupled spins, such as lactate methyl protons. Finally, STEAM allows for shorter TE values, reducing signal losses from T2 relaxation and allowing observation of metabolites with short T2.

12.2.2   Multiple Voxel Techniques

Multiple voxel techniques are those from which multiple spectra are obtained during a single measurement. The most common of these methods is known as *chemical shift imaging* (CSI). CSI techniques are analogous to standard imaging techniques in that phase encoding gradient tables are used for spatial localization. They are subdivided into 1D, 2D and 3D versions, depending on the number of gradient tables used for spatial localization. The most common of these approaches is 2D-CSI, in which two gradient tables are used. Volume selective rf excitation pulses are used, either with a PRESS or STEAM rf pulse train. The most common scheme has the three excitation pulses in mutually perpendicular directions and is termed *volume selective CSI* (Figure 12-4). This scheme enables the volume of excitation to be tailored so that areas producing contaminating signal can be avoided. For example, brain stud-

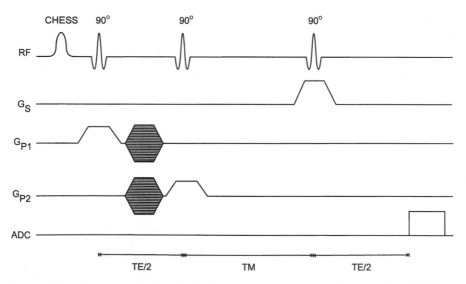

Figure 12-4. Volume selective 2D-CSI pulse sequence timing diagram. The CHESS rf pulse is used for suppression of water.

ies using volume selective CSI can minimize the signal from the skull and subcutaneous fat.

Volume selective CSI techniques have the advantage over SVS techniques in that spectra from several volumes of tissue can be measured simultaneously, which is advantageous if the disease under observation is diffuse or covers a large area of anatomy. However, the measurement times for CSI techniques are generally relatively long, and the entire data collection must be completed in order to obtain all the localization phase encoding steps. With SVS techniques, the measurement times are long due to multiple acquisitions necessary to produce adequate S/N, but the number of acquisitions can be adjusted depending on the voxel size. In addition, the multiple voxels must be individually postprocessed, making analysis of CSI data more operator intensive.

12.3   SPECTRAL ANALYSIS AND POSTPROCESSING

The MRS signal from a voxel contains information regarding the identity, molecular environment, and concentration of the metabolite producing the signal. This information is provided by the resonant frequency, the linewidth (full width at half maximum height), and the integrated peak area, respectively. Although this information could be extracted from the time domain form of the signal, it is more convenient to analyze the frequency domain form, obtained following a Fourier transformation. This analysis is aided by various data processing techniques applied both prior to and following the Fourier transformation (Figure 12-5). Many of these are often used in MRI techniques. Filtering of the echo signal is performed to reduce noise that can be induced during the very long sampling times for the echo (typically 1000 ms). This is the same type of filter used in MRI to reduce truncation artifacts. Zero filling consists of adding data points of zero amplitude to the end of the detected time domain signal. This data is typically background noise in the measurement. Following Fourier transformation, the frequency resolution of the resulting spectrum is increased through interpolation of the measured data points. This approach, termed *sinc interpolation* in MRI, provides a smoother appearance to the final spectrum. The final processing that is applied to the time domain signal is a correction for distortion from residual eddy currents. Eddy currents are produced as a result of the time-varying nature of the gradient pulses and result in fluctuating magnetic fields that distort the MR signal. The measurement hardware performs some type of eddy current compensa-

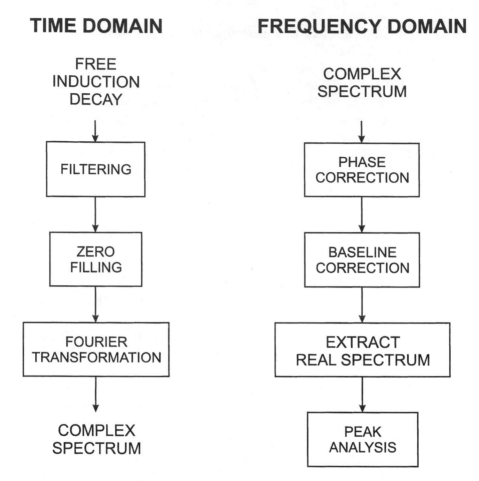

Figure 12-5. Typical postprocessing steps.

tion to correct for this as described in Chapter 13. While sufficient for MRI studies, this compensation is often insufficient to produce undistorted MR spectra. Acquisition of a second signal, usually a water-unsuppressed signal from the same voxel, is used to provide a reference for residual field variations due to eddy currents.

Following Fourier transformation, the resulting complex frequency domain signal is not a single mode signal, but is usually a mixture of both the in-phase (dispersion) and out-of-phase (absorption) information relative to the transmitter (Figure 12-6). In MRI studies, rather than separating these two signals, they are combined to form the magnitude image. For MRS studies, the pure absorption mode is preferred, due to its simpler spectra and to enable semiquantitative spectral analysis. A

a.

b.

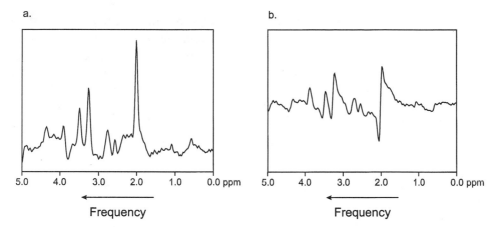

Frequency   Frequency

Figure 12-6. Phase-corrected complex spectrum resulting from Fourier transformation of FID signal. Measurement parameters are pulse sequence, STEAM; *TR*, 1500 ms; *TE*, 20 ms; number of sample points, 1024; number of acquisitions, 128; volume size, 20 × 20 × 20 mm³. (*a*) Real portion of spectrum, also known as the *absorption spectrum*; (*b*) Imaginary portion of spectrum, also known as the *dispersion spectrum*.

process known as *phase correction* is used to separate the two modes and extract the absorption portion. A mathematical manipulation combines the two components of the complex signal together in such a way as to isolate the absorption mode to the real portion and the dispersion mode to the imaginary portion. For the real spectrum, it may also be necessary to perform a baseline correction if it is not flat. It may not be flat due to hardware imperfections or incomplete water suppression. Finally, the resonant frequency, linewidth, and integrated area for each peak in the spectrum can be measured. Although a visual examination of the spectrum can provide an approximation of these parameters, the most accurate method for analysis involved fitting of the peaks to theoretical curves of the appropriate shape. Whereas the frequencies and linewidths can be compared directly from one spectrum to another, peak areas are influenced by various hardware-related variables that are difficult to quantify. Instead, ratios of peak areas are used in evaluating the relative concentrations of the metabolites. Absolute concentrations for metabolites can be determined if a simultaneous measurement of a reference compound is performed, in which the concentration of the reference is known by other means.

One example of a clinical application of MRS is in the evaluation of temporal lobe epilepsy. Normal brain spectra obtained with long *TE* (135 and 270 ms) show three major peaks: N-Acetyl aspartate (NAA) at 2.02

ppm, Creatine/phosphocreatine (Cr) at 3.0 ppm, and Choline (Cho) at 3.2 ppm relative to water at 4.7 ppm. The relative area ratios in adults are typically 1.4–1.5 for NAA/Cr and 0.8 for Cho/Cr. Patients with temporal lobe epilepsy have been found to have reduced levels of NAA and increased levels of Cho and Cr in the diseased lobe (Achten, 1997). Acquisition of spectra from both temporal lobes enables a clear identification of the affected region.

CHAPTER 13

Instrumentation

A very important aspect of MRI is the instrumentation used to produce the images. Many MR systems are commercially available, each possessing different features and capabilities. Many of these features are related to the operating software provided by the manufacturer, but certain hardware components are common to all systems. The following sections describe the basic subsystems of an MRI scanner and technical aspects to consider in comparing systems. The major components are a computer/array processor, a magnet system, a gradient system, a radio-frequency system, and a data acquisition system (Figure 13-1).

13.1   COMPUTER/ARRAY PROCESSOR

Currently, every MRI system has a minimum of two computers. The main, or host, computer controls the user interface software. This software enables the operator to directly or indirectly control all functions of the scanner. Scan parameters may be selected or modified, patient images may be displayed or recorded on film or other media, and post-processing such as region-of-interest measurements or magnification can be performed. Several peripheral devices are attached to the main computer. A hard disk is used to store the patient images immediately following reconstruction. This disk has limited capacity and is used for short-term storage. A device for long-term archival storage, either laser optical disk or magnetic tape, is usually included. A camera is also attached to the main computer if filming is controlled by the operating software.

One or more consoles are attached to the main computer. The console is the primary device for operator input. Each console has a keyboard and one or more monitors for displaying images and text information. Many systems use a computer mouse or trackball for more interactive control. The second and subsequent consoles may be directly attached to the same main computer or may be separate workstations that access the image data through a network connection.

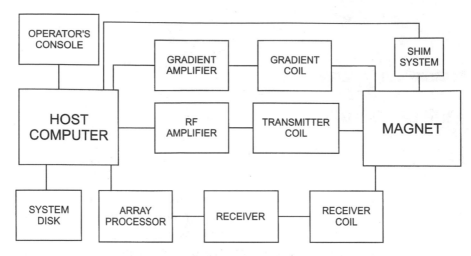

Figure 13-1. Block diagram of an MRI system.

An array processor is also part of a standard MRI system. It is a dedicated computer system used for performing the 2D Fourier transformation of the detected data. The array processor is controlled by the operating software. The raw data is stored from the receiver into memory in the array processor itself or onto a separate hard disk. The array processors currently used with MRI scanners are capable of performing the Fourier transformation for a 256 * 256 matrix in less than 1 second. Additional array processors may be present that perform computationally intensive postprocessing.

Many MRI systems are connected to additional computers using network connections, allowing images to be transferred from the MRI computer to another computer in a remote location. Two types of connections are common. One type is a physical cable, referred to as an *Ethernet connection*. This connection may be between two scanners, or between the scanner and a computer system known as a PACS (picture archiving and communications system) unit. This type of system can provide image transfer to physician viewing stations and/or long-term archiving of the digital images. Alternately, the connection may be through a dial-up modem, using standard or high-speed telecommunication. It is also important that the two computers are able to communicate with each other using a common language. Although not universally used, the industry standard for image transfer between computer systems is DICOM, which stands for digital imaging and communication in medicine. Images written using this format have the basic measurement information stored so that any vendor can read and properly display the images with the correct anatomic labeling and basic measurement parameters.

13.2   MAGNET SYSTEM

The magnet is the basic component of an MRI scanner. Magnets are available in a variety of field strengths, shapes, and materials. All magnet field strengths are measured in units of tesla or gauss (1 tesla = 10,000 gauss). Magnets are usually categorized as low, medium, or high field systems. Low-field magnets have main field strengths less than 0.5 T. Medium-field systems have main magnetic fields between 0.5 and 1.0 T, and high-field systems have fields of 1.0 T or greater.

Magnets are also characterized by the metal used in their composition. Permanent magnets are manufactured from metal that remains magnetic for extremely long periods of time (years). They can be solenoidal (tube shaped) or have a more open design. Permanent magnets have minimum maintenance costs because the field is always present. However, care must be taken to keep ferrous material away from the magnet. Such material will be attracted forcefully into the magnet and the magnetic field cannot be eliminated to allow its extraction. Another type of magnet is electromagnets in which the flow of electrical current through wire coils produces the magnetic field. Traditional electromagnets are made of copper wire wound in loops of various shapes. A water-cooled power supply provides a current source. The magnetic field is present as long as current flows through the magnet windings. Copper wire-based electromagnets are low-field systems and may be also solenoidal or open-type design. The most common type of magnets are solenoidal super-conducting magnets using niobium-titanium alloy wire immersed in liquid helium as the magnet wire. This alloy has no resistance to the flow of electrical current below a temperature of 20 K. The magnet cryostat, which contains the liquid helium, may be a double dewar design with a liquid nitrogen container surrounding the helium container, or a helium-only design with a refrigeration system to reduce the helium boiloff to a minimum. Refrigeration systems used with current magnets allow helium replenishment rates of 1−2 times per year.

The primary consideration in magnet quality is the homogeneity or uniformity of the magnetic field. Field homogeneity is usually expressed in ppm relative to the main field over a certain distance. Magnetic field values are measured at various locations inside the magnet and used to calculate the field variation using equation [2-4], replacing the frequencies with the measured magnetic field values. High homogeneity means the magnetic field changes very little over the specified region or volume. The protons in this region resonate at the same frequency and thus produce the maximum possible signal. Great effort is taken during magnet manufacturing and installation to ensure the best homogeneity possible. However, manufacturing imperfections or site problems (e.g., nearby steel posts, asymmetrical metal arrangements) may produce significant field distortions. To correct for this, the distortions are characterized by the shape of the field corrections required as a function of distance away from the magnet center. This classification is referred as the order of the field or shim correction used. First order or linear corrections in each direction are achieved using the imaging gradient coils described in Section 13.3. Second or higher order corrections are nonlinear in nature and most MRI systems use a coil known as a *shim coil* to correct for them. The design of the shim coil may be passive in that it holds pieces of metal (shim plates) or small magnets that correct the field distortions, or active in that there are loops of wire through which current passes to correct the field distortions. In some systems, both types of shim correction may be used. Passive shimming is generally performed at the time of magnet installation as a one-time event. Active shimming (also called *electrical shimming*) is usually performed on a regular basis during system maintenance. Field homogeneity is an important factor to consider when evaluating an MRI system.

Certain precautions should be exercised around all magnets, regardless of field strength. The examination room in which the magnet is located should have restricted access. Any metal near the magnet should be nonmagnetic. Metal items such as stethoscopes or pens may be attracted to the magnet, causing possible injury. Electrical equipment must be protected or shielded from the magnetic field in order to function properly. Patients with surgical implants or metal fragments in their bodies as a result of trauma or occupation (e.g., sheet metal workers) should be scanned only if there is no risk to the patient should the implant or fragment move during the procedure. Patients with pacemakers or ferromagnetic intracranial aneurysm clips should not be scanned under any circumstances due to the risk of patient injury. The magnetic properties of various medical implants have been extensively described by Shellock and coworkers (Shellock, 1998).

It is also important to realize that the magnetic field of all magnets extends in all directions away from the center of the field. The amount of fringe magnetic field, the portion outside the magnet housing, is a very important consideration in siting an MRI system. The fringe field is greatest near the magnet in the z direction and decreases with increasing distance away from the magnet. The fringe field is also larger for higher field magnets. A low-field magnet has a very small fringe field, making it easier to use standard patient monitoring equipment. High-field systems are often manufactured with magnetic shielding of some variety to reduce the fringe field. This shielding may surround the magnet (passive shielding), be generated by a second set of superconducting magnet windings opposing the main field (active shielding), or be built into the wall (room shielding). Two distances are of concern regarding the fringe field. The 0.5 mT (5 G) distance is considered the minimum safe distance for persons with pacemakers. This distance prevents interference of the pacemaker operation by the magnetic field. The 0.1 mT (1 G) distance, the nominal distance for other equipment that uses video monitors, prevents distortion of the image on the monitor by the magnetic field. The actual distances are installation and equipment specific. Contact the manufacturer regarding individual situations.

13.3   GRADIENT SYSTEM

As mentioned in Chapter 4, small linear distortions to B_0 known as gradient fields or gradients are used to localize the tissue signals. Three gradients are used, one each in the x, y, and z directions, to produce the orthogonal field distortions required for imaging. They are each generated by the flow of electrical current through separate loops of wire mounted into a single form known as the *gradient coil*. Variations in gradient amplitude are produced by changes in the amount or direction of the current flow through the coil.

One of the major criteria for evaluation of an MRI scanner is the capabilities of the gradient system. There are four aspects that are important in assessing gradient system performance: maximum gradient strength, rise time or slew rate, duty cycle, and techniques for eddy current compensation. Gradient strength is measured in units of mT m^{-1} or G cm^{-1} (1 G cm^{-1} = 10 mT m^{-1}), with typical maximum gradient strengths for current state-of-the-art MRI systems being 20–25 mT m^{-1} (2.0–2.5 G cm^{-1}). These maximum gradient strengths allow thinner slices or smaller FOV to be obtained without changing other measurement parameters.

The response of a gradient coil to the flow of current is not instantaneous. Gradient pulses require a finite time known as the rise time to achieve their final value. This rise time is nominally 0.5–1.0 ms, which defines a rate of change or slew rate for a gradient pulse. If the desired gradient pulse amplitude is 10 mT m^{-1} with a 1 ms rise time, the slew rate is 10 mT m^{-1} ms^{-1}. Gradient rise times and/or slew rates are often used to evaluate the performance of the gradient amplifier or power supply producing the current. High performance amplifiers allow shorter rise times/faster slew rates enabling shorter gradient pulse durations and/ or interpulse delays within a pulse sequence. As a result, the minimum echo time may be reduced for a given technique while maintaining a small FOV.

The duty cycle of the gradient amplifier is another important measure of gradient performance. The duty cycle determines how fast the amplifier can respond to the demands of a pulse sequence. Duty cycles of 100% at the maximum gradient amplitude are typical for state-of-the-art gradient amplifiers for normal imaging sequences. Large duty cycles allow high amplitude gradient pulses to be used with very short interpulse delays.

Another complication of gradient pulses is eddy currents. Eddy currents are electric fields produced in a conductive medium by a changing magnetic field. In MRI systems, eddy currents are typically induced by the ramping gradient pulse in the body coil located inside the gradient coil and the cryoshield (the innermost portion of the magnet cryostat) outside the coil. These currents generate a magnetic field that opposes and distorts the original gradient pulse. Because eddy currents are produced during the ramping of the pulse, they fluctuate with time and cause the distorting field to change with time as they decay. Therefore the magnetic field homogeneity and the corresponding frequencies change with time as well. Correction of these eddy current-induced distortions is known as *eddy current compensation*. Two approaches are commonly used for compensation. One method predistorts the gradient pulse so that the field variation inside the magnet is the desired one. This predistortion may be done via hardware or software. A second approach uses a second gradient coil surrounding the main gradient coil with windings in the opposite direction. This approach is called an *actively shielded gradient coil*, analogous to the actively shielded magnet described previously. The opposing current flow through the shield coil reduces the eddy currents induced outside the coil. Typical state-of-the-art scanners use both methods of eddy current compensation.

13.4   RADIOFREQUENCY SYSTEM

The rf transmitter system is responsible for generating and broadcasting the rf pulses used to excite the protons. The rf transmitter contains four main components: a frequency synthesizer, the digital envelope of rf frequencies, a high power amplifier, and a coil or antenna. As discussed in Chapter 4, each rf pulse has both a frequency and a phase defined for it. These features are determined by the combination of frequency and phase from the frequency synthesizer and the rf envelope defining the pulse shape.

The frequency synthesizer produces the center or carrier frequency for the rf pulse. It also provides the master clock for the measurement hardware during the scan. The frequency synthesizer also controls the relative phase of the rf pulse. Many pulse sequences alternate the phase of the excitation pulse for each measurement by 180° to help reduce stimulated echo artifacts caused by pulse imperfections. Spin echo sequences also typically have the refocusing rf pulses shifted in phase 90° relative to the excitation pulse (known as a Carr-Purcell-Meiboom-Gill or CPMG technique). This phase variation may be done through modulation of the rf envelope or of the carrier frequency. More sophisticated synthesizers allow phase changes of $1-2°$ increments. This finer control also allows for coherence spoiling through incremental phase change of the transmitter, a process known as *rf spoiling* (Chapter 8).

The rf envelope is stored as a discrete envelope or function containing a range or bandwidth of frequencies. It is mixed with the carrier frequency prior to amplification to produce an amplitude modulated pulse at the desired frequency. For some scanners, the final frequency is produced exclusively by the frequency synthesizer, while for other scanners, the rf envelope is modulated to incorporate a frequency offset into the pulse. In either case, the particular frequency is determined based on equation [4-1] and generated as a phase coherent signal by the synthesizer.

The rf power amplifier is responsible for producing sufficient power from the frequency synthesizer signal to excite the protons. The amplifier may be solid state or a tube type. Typical rf amplifiers for MR scanners are rated at $2-15$ kW of output power. The actual amount of power required from the amplifier to rotate the protons from equilibrium depends on the field strength, coil transmission efficiency, transmitter pulse duration, and desired excitation angle.

The final component of the rf system is the transmitter coil. All MR measurements require a transmitter coil or antenna to broadcast the rf signals. Although transmitter coils can be any size and shape, the one requirement that must be met is that they generate an effective $\mathbf{B}_1$ field perpendicular to $\mathbf{B}_0$. Another feature of most transmitter coils is that they can produce uniform rf excitation over a desired area; that is, a volume can be defined within the coil where all protons experience the same amount of rf energy. Solenoidal MR systems use a saddle coil design, which produces uniform rf excitation even though the coil opening is parallel to B_0. These coils are often adjusted or tuned to the patient to achieve the maximum efficiency in rf transmission.

Two types of coil polarity are used: linear polarized (LP) and circularly polarized (CP), also called *quadrature*. In an LP system, a single coil system is present and the rf pulse is broadcast as a plane wave. A plane wave broadcast at a frequency ω_{TR} has two circularly rotating components, rotating in opposite directions at the same frequency ω_{TR}. For MR, only the component rotating in the same direction as the protons (in-phase) induces resonance absorption. The other component (out-of-phase) is absorbed by the patient as heat. In a CP transmitter system, two coils are present, one rotated 90° from the other. Equivalent rf pulses are broadcast through each coil. The out-of-phase components cancel each other while the in-phase components add coherently. The patient absorbs only the energy from the in-phase components from each coil. A 40% improvement in efficiency from the transmitter system is achieved for a CP system relative to an equivalent LP system for the same proton rotation.

Although MR is considered a relatively safe imaging technique, the absorbed rf power generates heat inside the patient. In the United States, manufacturers are required by the Food and Drug Administration (FDA) to monitor the rf power absorbed by the patient so that excessive patient heating does not occur over both the excited tissue volume (localized) and the entire patient. To accomplish this, the specific absorption rate of energy dissipation or SAR is monitored. The SAR is measured in watts of energy per kilogram of patient body weight (W/kg). MRI systems are designed to operate at or below the SAR guidelines, which are set to limit the patient heating to approximately 1°C or less. For low-field scanners, the SAR seldom limits the measurement protocols. For high-field scanners, the SAR limits have a significant effect on the number of slices or saturation pulses that can be applied to the patient within a scan.

13.5 DATA ACQUISITION SYSTEM

The data acquisition system is responsible for measuring the signals from the protons and digitizing them for later postprocessing. All MRI systems use a coil to detect the induced voltage from the protons following an rf pulse. The coil is tuned to the particular frequency of the returning signal. This coil may be the same one used to broadcast the rf pulse, or it may be a dedicated receiver coil. The exact shape and size of the coil are manufacturer specific, but its effective field must be perpendicular to B_0. The sensitivity of the coil depends on its size, with smaller coils being more sensitive than larger coils. Also, the amount of tissue within the sensitive volume of the coil, known as the *filling factor*, affects the sensitivity. For large-volume studies such as body or head imaging, the transmitter coil often serves as the receiver coil. For smaller-volume studies, receive-only surface coils are usually used. These coils are small, usually ring-shaped, have high sensitivity but limited penetration, and are used to examine anatomy near the surface of the patient's body. Phased array coils use two or more smaller surface coils to cover a larger area. This arrangement provides the sensitivity of the small coil but with the anatomical coverage of the larger coil.

The signals produced by the protons are usually $nV-\mu V$ in amplitude and MHz in frequency. In order to process them, amplification is required, which is usually performed in several stages. The initial amplification is performed using a low noise, high-gain preamplifier located inside the magnet room or built into the coil itself. This signal is further amplified, demodulated to a kHz frequency, filtered using a low pass filter, and divided into the real and imaginary parts before being detected by the analog-to-digital converters (ADCs). The ADCs digitize each analog signal at a rate determined by the sampling time and number of data points specified by the user. Typical ADCs can digitize a 10-V signal into 16 bits of information at a rate of $0.5-1000$ μsec per data point. The digitized data is stored onto a hard disk or onto computer memory for later Fourier transformation. Phased array coils typically have a separate preamplifier and ADC for each coil in the array.

Although not formally part of the data acquisition system hardware, an important component of an MRI scanner is rf shielding of the scan room. The weak MR signals must be detected in the presence of background rf signals from local radio and television stations. To filter this extraneous noise, MRI scanners are normally enclosed in a copper or stainless steel shield known as a Faraday shield. Maintaining the integrity of this Faraday shield is very important to ensure minimal noise contamination of the final images.

13.6 SUMMARY OF SYSTEM COMPONENTS

Following is a list of variables to consider in comparing MRI systems according to subsystem:

Computer/Array Processor

Speed of main computer
Capacity of short-term storage disk, MBytes
Type of archive device
Number and speed of array processors, s image^{-1}
Number of consoles and method of interconnection
Network capability
DICOM compatibility

Magnet System

Field strength, T
Field homogeneity, ppm measured over a certain diameter of a spherical volume (dsv)
0.5 mT distance from isocenter, ft

Gradient System

Maximum gradient amplitude, mT m^{-1} (or G cm^{-1})
Duty cycle, in percent
Slew rate, mT m^{-1} ms^{-1}
Method(s) of eddy current correction

Radiofrequency System

Rf spoiling capabilities (phase behavior)
Maximum output power, kW
Type of transmitter coils (CP, LP)

Data Acquisition System

Speed, size, and maximum voltage of ADCs
Raw data storage capacity, MBytes
Types of receiver coils (CP, LP, phased array)
Nature and quality of rf shielding

CHAPTER 14

Contrast Agents

One of the strengths of MRI is the significant amount of intrinsic contrast between tissues. This contrast is based upon differences in signal intensity between adjacent pixels in the image. It is a result primarily of differences in the T1 and/or T2 relaxation times of the tissues under observation accentuated by the chosen *TR* and *TE*. Pathologic tissue may or may not have significant differences in T1 or T2 from the surrounding normal tissue. For this reason, there may be little contrast between normal and pathologic tissue in spite of the inherent high contrast in the images. Administration of a contrast agent can be used to increase this contrast.

Contrast agents for MRI have several advantages over those used for computed tomography (CT). CT agents are direct agents in that they contain an atom (iodine, barium) that attenuates or scatters the incident X-ray beam. This scattering permits direct visualization of the agent itself regardless of its location. MRI contrast agents are indirect agents in that they are never visualized directly in the image, but affect the relaxation times of the water protons in the nearby tissue. The concentration and dosage for MRI agents is also significantly lower than for CT agents, which in part explains the lower occurrence of adverse reactions to MRI agents. They are normally excreted through the renal system within three to four days, though the excretion half-time varies substantially from agent to agent. Contrast agents are usually categorized as T1 or T2 agents based on their primary effect of shortening the T1 or T2 relaxation times, respectively. However, these agents also shorten the other relaxation time to a lesser degree. The amount of reduction depends on the concentration of the agent; when concentrated, T1 agents shorten T2 or T2* times and when dilute, T2 agents reduce T1 times. Contrast agents may also be grouped into intravenous and oral agents depending on the route of administration. The following is a brief discussion of MR contrast agents with emphasis on those in current clinical use.

14.1 INTRAVENOUS AGENTS

14.1.1 T1 Relaxation Agents

Most intravenous contrast agents currently in clinical use are T1 relaxation agents. A variety of formulations are available, all of which consist of one or more paramagnetic metal ions that contain one or more unpaired electrons. The metal ions are bound into a chelate complex or contained within a macromolecule. The relaxation efficiency per molecule depends on several factors, including the size of the metal-chelate complex and the nature of the metal ion. The primary mode of operation for T1 contrast agents is as a relaxation sink for the water protons. As mentioned in Chapter 3, T1 relaxation depends upon the "lattice" receiving the energy that the protons have absorbed from the rf excitation pulse. This energy transfer occurs most efficiently when the protons are in the innermost layer of atoms surrounding the metal ion, known as the *coordination sphere*. Because the chelate molecules are relatively large and have many bonds to the metal ion, there is limited free space in the coordination sphere, which prevents the protons on large molecules such as fat from getting sufficiently close to the metal ion for efficient energy transfer. The tissue water is able to diffuse into the coordination sphere of the metal ion and give up its energy, then exchange with the bulk tissue water, enabling additional water molecules to enter the coordination sphere. This diffusion/exchange happens very rapidly ($\sim 10^6$ times per second) so that the bulk tissue water is relaxed when the subsequent excitation pulse is applied (Figure 14-1). The result is that the tissue signal near the contrast agent is much greater than for the neighboring tissue in a T1-weighted image. In addition, the rapid exchange process enables many water molecules to be affected by a single chelate complex, which allows low concentrations of contrast agent to be used in clinical studies.

Intravenous T1 contrast agents are available in both ionic and nonionic formulations. The most common agents use gadolinium as the metal ion and either diethyenetriaminepentaacetate (DPTA) [ionic: Magnevist; Schering AG, Berlin, Germany], diethylenetriaminepentaacetate bismethylamide [nonionic: Omniscan; Nycomed, Oslo, Norway] or 10-(2-hydroxypropyl)-1,4,7,10-tetraazacyclododecane-1,4,7-triacetate (HP-DO3A) [nonionic: Prohance; Bracco, Princeton, New Jersey] as the chelate molecule. The agents currently licensed for use in the United States are nonspecific extracellular agents, in that the agents diffuse rapidly from the vascular space into the interstitial space of the tissue (see Figure 11-3). The major elimination pathway of these agents is through glo-

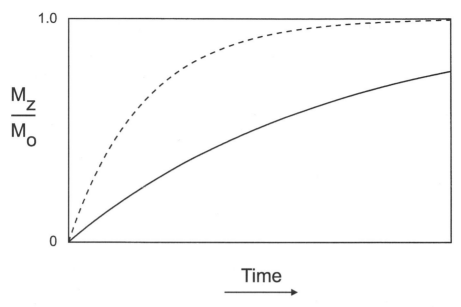

Figure 14-1. T1 recovery curves for tissue in the absence (solid line) and in the presence (dashed line) of T1 relaxation agent. In the presence of the agent, the T1 relaxation time for the tissue water is shortened, so that the net magnetization for the "enhanced" tissue becomes significantly greater. More signal is measured from the enhanced tissue in all cases.

merular filtration and renal excretion. The half life in humans is typically in the order of 90 minutes with virtually complete elimination of these agents within 24 hours. The safety profile for these agents is excellent, with few reported side effects and rare cases of major side effects. These agents are therefore frequently employed in patients with a known history of allergies to iodinated contrast agents. In addition, these agents are considered to be extremely safe for administration to patients with compromised renal function, due to both the intrinsic safety of these agents and the relatively small volume of the agent administered for most studies (typically 10 to 20 ml). On the other hand, the adverse effect of iodinated contrast in patients with renal failure is a well-known problem. Therefore, patients with renal failure or elevated levels of serum creatinine are more likely to tolerate an MRI examination with gadolinium-chelate contrast administration rather than a CT examination with iodinated contrast media.

Newer formulations of gadolinium-chelate contrast agents have both hydrophilic and hydrophobic properties. Examples of these include benzoxypropionic tetraacetate (BOPTA) and ethoxybenzyl diethylenetriaminepentaacetate (EOB-DTPA) as the ligand. The presence of a hydrophobic ligand enables hepatocyte uptake of these agents and elimination by the biliary system, rather than strictly through renal excretion. Approximately 10% of Gd-BOPTA [Multihance; Bracco, Princeton, New Jersey] is eliminated by the hepatobiliary system and 90% by renal excretion, whereas 50% of Gd-EOB-DTPA [Eovist; Schering AG, Berlin, Germany] is eliminated by the hepatobiliary system and 50% by renal excretion. The combined pathway of elimination for these agents enables both early postcontrast imaging, emphasizing tissue perfusion, and late postcontrast imaging, reflecting hepatocellular uptake and bile duct elimination. These agents are currently not licensed for clinical use in the United States; however, the combined effect of their ease of use, safety, and dual-phase behavior suggest that they have great potential as liver contrast agents.

Another metal ion that has been formulated into a T1 contrast agent for liver imaging is manganese. Manganese ion chelated to N,N'-dipyridoxal ethylenediamine-N,N'-diacetate 5,5' bis (phosphate) (Mn-DPDP) [Teslascan; Nycomed, Oslo, Norway] is a T1-weighted contrast agent that is hepatocyte-selective but is also absorbed by other organs and tissues including pancreas, and adrenal and renal cortex. Approximately 70% of the agent is eliminated by the hepatobiliary system and 30% by the urinary system. Mn-DPDP is administered via a slow intravenous injection over 1 to 2 minutes. This agent has a long imaging window with maximal hepatic parenchymal enhancement lasting from 15 minutes to 4 hours. The major clinical indication for the use of Mn-DPDP is in the determination of the extent of liver metastases in patients under consideration for surgical resection. Mn-DPDP may also be used to characterize liver lesions as hepatocyte-containing versus nonhepatocyte-containing and to improve delineation of pancreatic tumors (Figure 14-2). Adverse reactions are relatively uncommon with this agent.

Other T1 contrast agents have been developed using gadolinium chelated to macromolecules or polymers. These agents remain within the blood stream rather than diffuse into the tissue. Their use as MR angiographic agents and as agents to assess the integrity of capillary basement membrane is currently under investigation.

14.1.2   T2 Relaxation Agents

The other class of intravenous contrast agents are T2 relaxation agents. They are typically macromolecules containing several iron atoms that

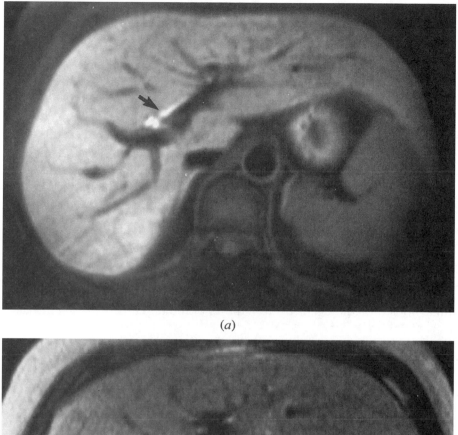

(a)

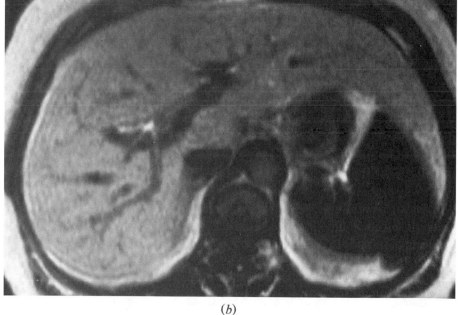

(b)

Figure 14-2. T1-weighted spoiled gradient echo images of liver following administration of Mn-DPDP contrast agent. Increased biliary excretion of Mn is demonstrated by the increased signal (arrows). (a) Fat suppression pulse is applied. (b) No fat suppression is used.

form a superparamagnetic center. The large magnetic susceptibility of the macromolecule distorts the local magnetic field in the vicinity of the agent, causing the nearby water protons to dephase more rapidly than the surrounding tissue. This condition results in significant signal loss in T2-weighted spin echo or gradient echo images. The most common T2 contrast agents are based on superparamagnetic iron oxide (SPIO) particulate molecules, also known as *ferumoxides*. These agents are selectively absorbed by the reticulo-endothelial cells located in the liver, spleen, and bone marrow. Normal tissue in these organ systems take up the agent and have low signal on T2 or T2* weighted images. Lesions that do not contain reticulo-endothelial cells in appreciable numbers do not take up the agent and remain unaffected and therefore have relatively high signal (Figure 14-3).

Currently, the only T2 contrast agent licensed for clinical use in the United States is Feridex [magnetite-dextran; Schering AG, Berlin, Germany]. It is usually administered as a slow drip infusion over 30 minutes. A further delay of 30 minutes prior to imaging allows for maximal uptake of the agent by reticulo-endothelial cells. This agent has a

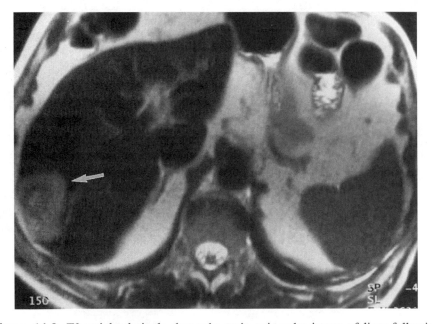

Figure 14-3. T2-weighted single-shot echo train spin echo image of liver following administration of superparamagnetic iron oxide contrast agent. The T2 relaxation times of the normal tissue are reduced by the iron oxide, while the metastatic lesion shows less agent uptake.

long imaging window from 30 minutes to 4 hours post infusion. Feridex has a good safety profile, but has a potential side effect of acute back pain developing during contrast infusion, occurring in less than 3% of patients. This side effect is usually self-limiting and disappears when the infusion is stopped or slowed. The most important clinical indication for Feridex is in the determination of the extent of liver metastases in patients under consideration for surgical resection. This agent can also distinguish between hepatic origin tumors that contain reticulo-endothelial cells and tumors that do not. Resovist [magnetite/maghemite-carboxydextran; Schering AG, Belin, Germany] is a newer formulation of a ferumoxide agent that can be administered in a small dose by bolus injection. The advantage of this agent is ease of administration and the lack of back pain as a side effect. Resovist is currently under consideration for approval by the U.S. FDA. SPIO agents formulated to a smaller particle size than used for liver imaging are under investigation as contrast agents for the examination of lymph nodes. Normal or hyperplastic lymph nodes take up the agent and lose signal on T2-weighted images, whereas malignant lymph nodes do not take up the agent and therefore appear relatively high signal. Iron oxide particles have also been used to label monoclonal antibodies targeted to specific tissues receptor sites. Asioglycan protein receptor contrast agents are one example that is under development.

14.2   ORAL AGENTS

Oral contrast agents typically are nonspecific agents. The most common usage of them is in abdominal and pelvic studies to provide reliable differentiation of bowel from adjacent structures and to provide better delineation of bowel wall processes. Oral agents may be categorized as positive or negative agents. Positive agents increase the overall signal intensity within the image, generally by shortening the T1 and T2 relaxation times of tissue water. These agents are generally solutions of paramagnetic metal ions or metal-chelate complexes. Many of these agents are present in naturally occurring products (manganese in green tea and blueberry juice) or in over-the-counter medications (ferric ammonium citrate; Geritol; Beecham, Bristol, Tennessee). Other agents have been specifically formulated for use with MRI such as Lumenhance (manganese chloride; Bracco, Princeton, New Jersey) and Magnevist Enteral (gadolinium-DTPA; Schering AG, Berlin, Germany) as T1 relaxation agents and OMR (ferric ammonium citrate; Oncomembrane,

Seattle, Washington) as a T2 relaxation agent. Positive agents can provide excellent delineation of the bowel, but the increased signal may induce greater artifacts as a result of respiratory motion or peristalsis.

The other type of oral contrast agent is a negative agent. Negative agents eliminate signal from the tissue in the area of interest. Two approaches are used for negative agents. One is to reduce the T2 relaxation times using suspensions of ferumoxide particles. The particles may be suspended in aqueous solution (Ferumoxsil; Advanced Magnetics, Cambridge, Massachusetts) or adsorbed onto a polymer. The other approach is to have an agent that contains no protons, and therefore produces no visible MR signal. The most common agent of this type is Perflubron (perfluorooctylbromide [PFOB]; Alliance Pharmaceutical, San Diego, California). Barium sulfate, clay, and air have also been used for intraluminal studies. One significant problem with many negative contrast agents is that they increase the local magnetic susceptibility, which may induce significant dephasing artifacts at high field strengths.

CHAPTER 15

Clinical Applications

In selecting pulse sequences and measurement parameters for a specific application, MRI allows the user tremendous flexibility to produce variations in contrast between normal and diseased tissue. This flexibility is available when imaging both stationary tissue as well as flowing blood. For example, the use of both bright blood and dark blood MRA techniques described in Chapter 10 permits more accurate assessment of vascular patency and intravascular mass lesions. A typical patient examination acquires images with multiple types of contrast, providing the clinician with more complete information on the nature of the tissue under observation and increasing the likelihood of lesion detection. Imaging protocols commonly employ a combination of T1- and T2-weighted sequences because they generally achieve this objective. It is important the MR examinations be tailored to the organ(s) under investigation, the type of disease process and the individual patient. The MR physician may choose to provide detailed measurement parameters for each examination, or have a predetermined regimen of scans that are to be performed by a technologist. Establishing fixed measurement protocols ensure the efficient operation of the MR scanner and that reliable, reproducible imaging examinations are acquired.

15.1 GENERAL PRINCIPLES OF CLINICAL MR IMAGING

The fundamental principles of diagnostic MRI of the entire body are good and reproducible image quality, good visualization of disease processes, and comprehensive imaging information. Because ideal achievement of all three goals may not be practical, the proper choice of pulse sequences and/or measurement parameters can provide adequate results within a clinically acceptable scan time. In particular, the visualization of disease can be dramatically affected by the measurement protocol. The conspicuity of disease usually benefits by changing the signal of background tissue to be distinctly different from the disease process under investigation. For example, variation of the signal of fat by the use of fat nonsuppressed and fat suppressed sequences aids in the detection of lymph nodes. On T1-weighted images, lymph nodes have low signal and therefore are conspicuous in a background of high signal fat, while on T2-weighted images, lymph nodes are relatively bright and their conspicuity is improved by decreasing the signal of background fat using fat suppression techniques. Following administration of a gadolinium-chelate contrast agent, lymph nodes have significantly shorter T1 values and produce high signal on T1-weighted images. The use of fat suppression is helpful to reduce the competing high signal of fat. The combined use of gadolinium-chelate contrast agents and fat suppression to increase signal of diseased tissue and to decrease signal of background fat, respectively, is widely used in various organ systems including the orbits, the bony skeleton, soft tissue of the extremities, and the breast.

An additional consideration is that fat suppressed spoiled gradient echo may be preferable to fat suppressed spin echo when concomitant evaluation of patency of vessels is desired as in imaging vascular grafts for patency or infection, or for imaging extremities to assess soft tissue infection or vascular thrombosis. This is because spoiled gradient echo images acquired within 2 minutes following gadolinium-chelate administration display patent vessels with high signal intensity while spin echo images may have a signal void from both patent and thrombosed vessels. Flow is commonly seen as signal void on spin echo due to the dephasing of moving spins during the gradient pulses, while blood clot is low signal due to the presence of fibrinous clot and the $T2^*$ effects of blood break down products.

It is important when defining protocols for MRI studies to obtain a sufficient variety of sequences to provide comprehensive information, while at the same time not to be too redundant and generate excessively long exams. For example, our approach for imaging of the abdomen has been to employ a variety of short duration T1- and T2-weighted sequences with the majority of them performed in the transverse plane, but also obtain at least one set of images in a plane orthogonal to the transverse plane. The particular choice of planes for a measurement is dictated by the area of anatomy under observation.

15.2   EXAMINATION DESIGN CONSIDERATIONS

The initial studies of MRI used primarily transverse T1- and T2-weighted spin echo techniques. As the modality has matured, it has become clear that imaging strategies must be modified beyond this elementary approach. There are several reasons for this:

Imaging of organs in the plane of the best anatomical display. Imaging of the spine or the female pelvis requires the use of both sagittal and transverse images to best demonstrate the anatomical structures. Similarly, the evaluation of large masses in the region of the upper poles of the kidneys is facilitated by sagittal as well as transverse images. On the other hand, coronal images are useful for visualization of the left lobe of the liver.

Compensation for the most severe artifacts generated by various organ systems. Abdominal imaging is severely compromised by respiratory artifacts. Imaging protocols that employ breathhold spoiled gradient echo sequences (e.g., FLASH, spoiled GRASS) as described in Chapter 9 can produce images with substantial T1-weighting while minimizing respiratory artifacts. Cardiac gating is essential when imaging the thorax in order to minimize phase artifacts from cardiac motion.

Increased spatial resolution and/or signal-to-noise. Imaging of small anatomical regions such as extremities (e.g., ankles, wrists, knees) or the breast require specialized surface coils to maximize both signal-to-noise and spatial resolution.

The use of contrast agents. Imaging of nonorgan-deforming focal lesions in the liver, spleen, and pancreas using intravenous gadolinium chelate complexes requires rapid, breathhold imaging techniques to capture the capillary phase of lesion enhancement. This approach necessitates the use of spoiled gradient echo techniques (e.g., FLASH or spoiled GRASS) with temporal resolution of less than 20 seconds. In many instances, the visualization of contrast enhancement in T1-weighted images may be improved through the use of fat suppression to remove the competing high signal from fat.

15.3   PROTOCOL CONSIDERATIONS FOR ANATOMICAL REGIONS

The following considerations and recommendations are offered for imaging various organs systems. Exact sequence protocols are not provided because different manufacturers have different imaging capabilities and functions.

15.3.1 Brain

A number of innovations have been developed for brain examinations. These include magnetization transfer suppression (used for background water suppression), diffusion-weighted imaging (acute stroke), ETSE, fat suppression, MRA (vascular disease), FLAIR, and contrast agent enhancement using gadolinium-chelate complexes. Despite the advancements, the standard for MR examinations of the brain remains sagittal T1-weighted spin echo and transverse T1- and T2-weighted conventional spin echo (Figures 15-1, 15-2, 15-3). Thin-slice (3 mm) coronal images provide excellent visualization of the pituitary gland and sella tursica. Replacement of T2-weighted conventional spin echo with ETSE is often done with little loss in diagnostic content. Routine use of a T1 contrast agent in the investigation of neoplastic disease is recommended. Many centers use MRA techniques regularly in the investigation of cerebrovascular disease.

15.3.2 Neck

The use of a surface coil for neck imaging is essential due to the small volume of tissue. High resolution T1- and T2-weighted spin echo sequences are useful for visualizing soft tissue. The use of gadolinium-

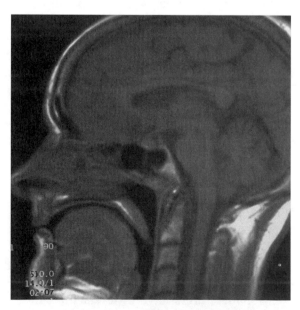

Figure 15-1. Sagittal spin echo T1-weighted head image. *TR*, 500 ms; *TE*, 15 ms.

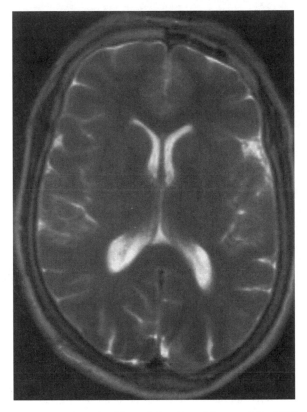

Figure 15-2. Transverse spin echo T2-weighted head image. *TR*, 2500 ms; *TE*, 90 ms.

chelate contrast agents may be helpful for tumor and lymph node detection, and for thyroid and parathyroid studies. The addition of fat suppression to postcontrast studies is helpful to delineate tissue. Uniform fat suppression may be difficult to achieve because of magnetic field distortions from the large magnetic susceptibility differences between the neck and the upper thorax.

15.3.3 Spine

A combination of T1- and T2-weighted images is important. Both sagittal and transverse images are valuable for examining the spinal cord and structural deformations such as disk herniations (Figures 15-4, 15-5, 15-6). Transverse images allow excellent visualization of nerve roots and possible disk fragments. Use of spatial presaturation pulses is recommended to reduce artifacts from jaw motion in cervical studies or abdominal motion in lumbar studies. Gadolinium-chelate contrast ad-

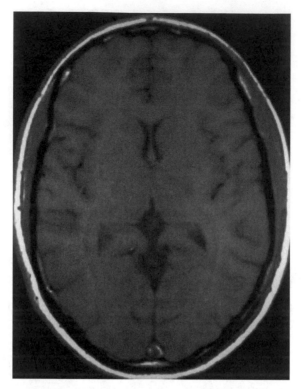

Figure 15-3. Transverse spin echo T1-weighted head image, *TR*, 500 ms; *TE*, 15 ms.

ministration and fat suppression are recommended in circumstances in which bony metastases are suspected.

15.3.4 Musculoskeletal

A combination of T1- and T2-weighted images is routinely used in musculoskeletal imaging. Images should be acquired in at least two orthogonal planes to ensure proper anatomical visualization (Figures 15-7, 15-8, 15-9). STIR images are frequently valuable for detection of tumor, inflammation, or avascular necrosis and may replace T2-weighted images in some settings. T2*-weighted images are often used for visualizing fluid and bony detail. Use of gadolinium-chelate contrast agents is important for the evaluation of inflammatory and neoplastic disease, often in combination with fat suppression. When imaging small anatomical regions away from the magnet isocenter, field homogeneity may limit the usefulness of fat suppression.

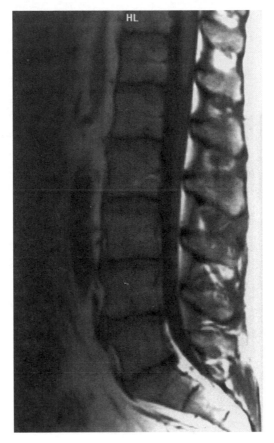

Figure 15-4. Sagittal spin echo T1-weighted lumbar spine image. *TR*, 500 ms; *TE*, 15 ms. Anterior spatial presaturation pulse is used to suppress peristalsis and respiration artifacts.

15.3.5 Thorax

Transverse T1-weighted spin echo images provide adequate anatomical perspective in the thoracic area. Cardiac triggering is essential to minimize motion artifacts from the heart. T2-weighted transverse images are helpful, particularly in the evaluation of chest wall or mediastinal involvement with cancer. T1-weighted images acquired with gadolinium-chelate contrast agents provides similar and complementary information. Fat suppression is a useful adjunct when gadolinium-chelate is employed. The lowered signal of fat improves the visualization of abnormal tissue enhancement, which is helpful for delineating the presence of chest wall invasion by malignant or infectious processes. Lesions in the

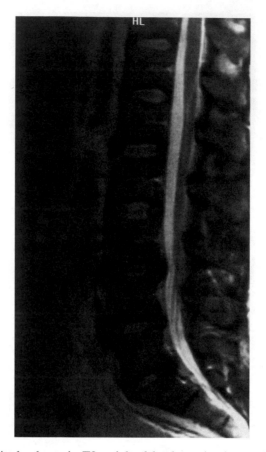

Figure 15-5. Sagittal echo train T2-weighted lumbar spine image. *TR*, 4000 ms; Effective *TE*, 90 ms; echo train length, 5. Anterior spatial presaturation pulse is used to suppress peristalsis and respiration artifacts.

lung apex and occasionally lung base require additional coronal or sagittal views. Breathhold imaging with gadolinium-chelate contrast enhancement improves visualization of small peripheral lung lesions such as metastases, which can be reliably seen at a diameter of 5 mm using this approach. For most examinations, imaging between 2 and 5 minutes following contrast administration provides a good balance of contrast enhancement of lung masses with diminished enhancement of the blood pool.

15.3.6   Breast

Optimal breast MR examination requires a dedicated breast coil to maximize spatial resolution. T1-weighted images following gadolinium-

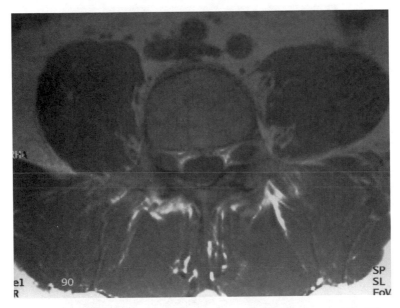

Figure 15-6. Transverse spin echo T1-weighted lumbar spine image. *TR*, 500 ms; *TE*, 15 ms.

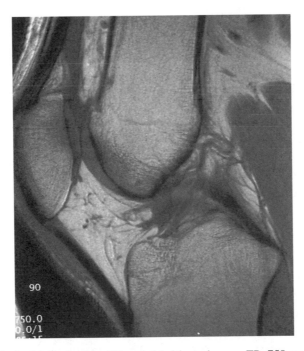

Figure 15-7. Sagittal spin echo T1-weighted knee image. *TR*, 750 ms; *TE*, 20 ms.

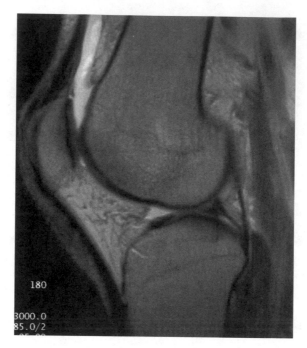

Figure 15-8. Sagittal echo train T2-weighted knee image. *TR*, 3000 ms; Effective *TE*, 85 ms; echo train length, 5.

chelate contrast administration are important for detection of lesions. Thin section, 3D-volume acquisition, rapid imaging, image subtraction, and application of techniques to reduce fat signal (fat saturation, water excitation, STIR) are important considerations for protocol development. Serial, dynamic imaging following gadolinium-chelate administration provides useful information on lesion characterization (see Figure 11-4). Many cancers enhance in an early intense fashion while most benign disease processes enhance in a delayed, less intense fashion. Further information regarding lesion morphology may be provided using high resolution T2-weighted ETSE sequences.

15.3.7   Heart and Great Vessels

Transverse cardiac-triggered T1-weighted spin echo sequences are essential in the evaluation of cardiac anatomy. High spatial resolution is frequently needed, particularly in assessing congenital heart disease; therefore, a slice thickness of less than 5 mm is recommended. Coronal and sagittal cardiac-triggered T1-weighted images may provide additional information in many instances. They are essential in the evaluation

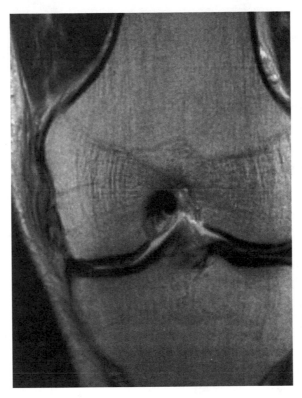

Figure 15-9. Coronal echo train spin echo T2-weighted knee image. *TR*, 3000 ms; *TE* 85 ms.

of congenital heart disease by providing anatomical information regarding vessels, airways, and cardiac chambers. The left anterior oblique sagittal plane is an important view for the evaluation of the thoracic aorta.

Signal from flowing blood within the cardiac chambers is often heterogeneous as a result of changes in flow direction and velocity. In spin echo sequences, it is helpful to minimize the signal from blood, both to reduce flow artifacts and to delineate vessels (dark blood techniques). Application of superior and inferior presaturation pulses or gradient dephasing may be required. Gradient motion rephasing should be avoided because it results in an increase signal from flowing blood. Alternately, techniques that result in high signal from flowing blood (bright blood techniques) are often helpful for the evaluation of chamber dynamics. Multiphasic techniques (cine MR) are particularly useful in the evaluation of wall motion and thickening, valvular disease and shunts. Useful projections include sagittal plane for pulmonary valve, coronal and left ventricular long axis for aortic valve, and transverse plane for tricuspid and mitral valves, and atrial and ventricular septal defects. On occasion, techniques with subsecond temporal resolution can minimize cardiac motion artifacts and are useful as dark blood techniques. For the evaluation of the aorta and major branches, a widely used technique is MR angiography employing a dynamic 3D gradient echo sequence following gadolinium-chelate administration.

15.3.8 Liver

T1- and T2-weighted transverse images are important for evaluating the liver. Combining breathhold and nonbreathhold sequences is often useful since some patients can hold their breath well but cannot breathe regularly, while others breathe regularly but cannot hold their breath well. More current protocols combine breathhold T1- and T2-weighted sequences with breathing independent T2-weighted sequences (Figures 15-10, 15-11, 15-12). A spoiled gradient echo sequence is most often used for T1-weighted imaging; however, T1-weighted spin echo with respiratory compensation may be considered for some patients. For T2-weighted images, breathing averaged ETSE with fat suppression is a useful technique. Performed as an echo train sequence, imaging time is

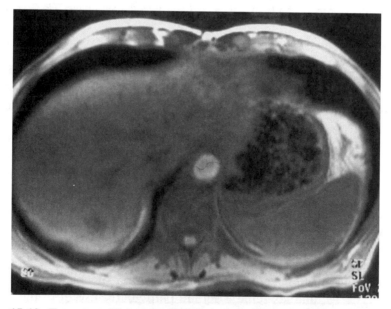

Figure 15-10. Transverse T1-weighted spoiled gradient echo liver image. *TR*, 170 ms; *TE*, 4 ms; flip angle, 80°.

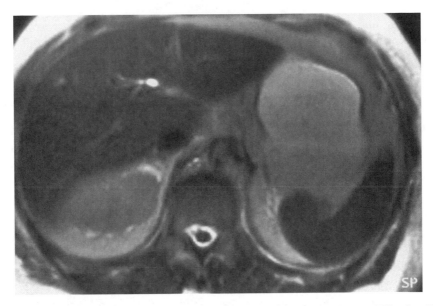

Figure 15-11. Transverse single shot echo train T2-weighted liver image. Effective *TE*, 90 ms.

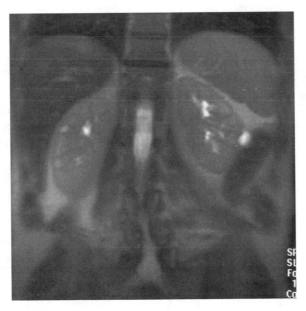

Figure 15-12. Coronal single shot echo train T2-weighted image of liver and kidneys. Effective *TE*, 90 ms.

reduced, and the addition of fat suppression diminishes respiratory ghosts, removes chemical shift artifacts, and diminishes the signal of a fatty infiltrated liver, which permits good visualization of the liver capsular surface and facilitates lesion detection.

The use of intravenous contrast agents improves lesion detection over nonenhanced imaging techniques. Currently available contrast agents include gadolinium-chelates and Mn-DPDP for T1 enhancement, and ferumoxides for T2 enhancement. When using gadolinium-chelate agents, it is important to image early after contrast (<30 seconds) to maximize the specific enhancement features of various focal hepatic lesions (Figure 15-13). Spoiled gradient echo techniques are extremely useful to accomplish this goal. In addition, serial sequence repetition with additional acquisitions at approximately 1 and 5 minutes may be routinely useful to visualize the temporal behavior of contrast uptake. Mn-DPDP has a longer imaging window (30 minutes–4 hours) so it lacks dynamic contrast enhancement ability. Unlike with gadolinium-chelate, it is not essential that the patient be able to suspend requisition to obtain a breath-hold spoiled gradient echo sequence because dynamic imaging is not

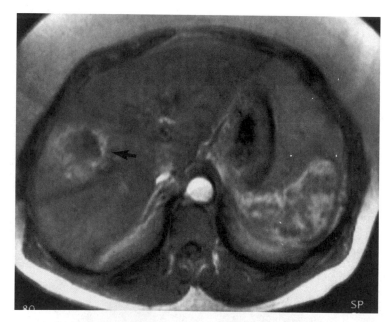

Figure 15-13. Transverse T1-weighted spoiled gradient echo liver image. *TR*, 170 ms; *TE*, 4 ms; flip angle, 90°. Immediately following gadolinium-chelate contrast administration, a lesion shows ring enhancement characteristic of metastatic colon cancer (arrow).

performed. High resolution (512 matrix) spoiled gradient echo is a useful sequence in combination with Mn-DPDP in that it permits detection of smaller focal lesions in conjunction with the T1-shortening effect of the agent. Fat suppression is another useful modification to employ with Mn-DPDP with the fat suppression serving to maximize the conspicuity of contrast enhancement (Figure 15-14). This may be particularly beneficial for imaging the pancreas.

Like Mn-DPDP, Feridex also has a long imaging window of 30 minutes–4 hours, and does not require the patient be able to suspend respiration. When using a ferumoxide agent, an important consideration for the choice of sequence is the dosage of iron administered. In Europe, a dose of iron is used that is one and one half times that of the dose used in North America. This higher dosage permits a greater choice of sequences that may be effective, including gradient echo sequences that are fundamentally T1-weighted. Care must be exercised in extrapolating information from European studies to American studies particularly in regard to sequence use. Sequences that are useful in conjunction with ferumoxide agents include fat suppressed ETSE, snap shot ETSE, echo train STIR, and gradient echo sequences with a relatively long TE and relatively low flip angle (e.g., $TR = 150$ ms, $TE = 9$ ms, flip angle =

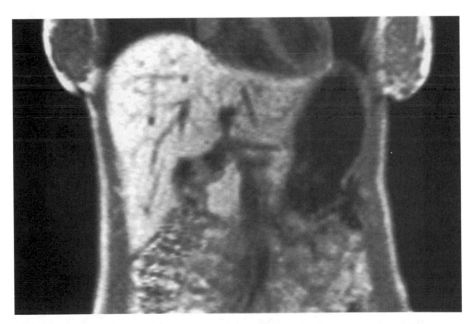

Figure 15-14. Coronal magnetization prepared T1-weighted liver image. Effective TE, 30 ms. Image is acquired following administration of Mn-DPDP.

45°). Examining for fatty infiltration requires out-of-phase gradient echo images prior to contrast administration.

15.3.9   Abdominal Organs

T1-weighted breathhold spoiled gradient echo and T1-weighted fat suppressed spin echo are both useful for controlling respiratory artifacts in the abdomen. As with the liver, combining breathhold with breathing independent sequences are advantageous. Snapshot ETSE T2-weighted sequences are particularly effective at demonstrating bowel and for distinguishing bowel from other entities. Transverse fat suppressed and conventional spoiled gradient echo images are useful in combination both prior to and following administration of intravenous gadolinium-chelate contrast agents. Following contrast administration, the unsuppressed technique is useful to provide capillary phase information while the subsequent acquisition of the fat suppressed technique provides interstitial phase information. Imaging of the adrenal glands require noncontrast out-of-phase gradient echo images.

15.3.10   Pelvis

Transverse images are routinely used, while sagittal images are a useful adjunct. T1-weighted images are frequently best performed as conventional spin echo or spoiled gradient echo, whereas T2-weighted images may be acquired as breathing averaged ETSE or snapshot ETSE. Thin slices (5 mm thickness) in the sagittal plane are necessary to optimally visualize the uterus and ovaries in the female and the seminal vesicles in the male. Gadolinium-chelate contrast administration is important in the evaluation of uterine and adnexal masses. Fat suppression is an important adjunct to contrast administration when ovarian cancer is clinically suspected.

15.4   RECOMMENDATIONS FOR SPECIFIC SEQUENCES AND CLINICAL SITUATIONS

15.4.1   T1-Weighted Techniques

Single Echo Spin Echo. For routine T1-weighted imaging, a moderate *TR* is recommended (400–700 ms at 1.0 and 1.5 T) with a short *TE* (20 ms or less). This combination allows acquisition of a sufficient number of slices yet provides acceptable contrast between gray and white matter. The slice thickness and in-plane spatial resolution can be tailored to the particular anatomical region under examination.

Spoiled Gradient Echo. Imaging parameters should include a relatively long *TR* ($\geq$140 ms) and the shortest in-phase echo time (4.5 ms at 1.5 T, 6.67 ms at 1.0 T), one acquisition and an excitation angle 70°–90°. These parameters maximize the number of slices, S/N, and T1-weighting, and minimize artifacts and the measurement time. This spoiled gradient echo sequence is ideal for T1-weighted imaging in the abdomen, for imaging in multiple planes, and for imaging following intravenous gadolinium-chelate contrast administration. When thin sections and high spatial resolution are desired and respiratory artifacts are not a problem, T1-weighted spin echo may be preferred.

Out-of-Phase Gradient Echo. Imaging parameters should include the shortest possible *TE*, preferably shorter than the in-phase *TE* (2.25 ms at 1.5 T, 3.3 ms at 1.0 T). This technique is best used to detect the presence of fat and water in similar proportions within a tissue volume. For clinical use, the most important applications for this technique are the examination for fatty infiltration of liver and for benign adenoma. In both entities, the observation of signal drop on out-of-phase images compared to in-phase images permits the diagnosis of fatty infiltration. For adrenal glands, this technique is virtually pathognomonic for benign disease in which the signal loss is uniform.

Fat Saturation. This technique is ideal when decreased phase artifact and expanded range of soft tissue signal intensities is desired. Improved demonstration of tissue with a high protein content (e.g., normal pancreas) or detection of subacute blood are important roles for T1-weighted fat saturation techniques. Following gadolinium-chelate contrast administration, the removal of the high signal intensity of fat results in easier discrimination of diseased tissue (e.g., diseased bowel or peritoneum, breast cancer, musculoskeletal neoplasms or inflammation). Fat-suppressed spin echo or spoiled gradient echo is also useful in the identification of fat composition in certain masses such as adrenal myelolipoma, colonic lipoma, or ovarian dermoid cyst. Unlike out-of-phase gradient echo techniques in which the maximal signal loss occurs in tissues where the fat and water are of equal proportions, fat suppression is most effective when the fat content in the tissue approaches 100%.

STIR. Musculoskeletal imaging benefits from the use of STIR imaging because of the relatively high signal from disease tissue. Images resemble those obtained by fat-suppressed T2-weighted spin echo techniques. STIR is not as sensitive to field homogeneity as fat saturation, and therefore is well suited for imaging small anatomical regions or away from the magnet isocenter. STIR sequences acquired with T1 times for fat and for silicon suppression are useful for the investigation of breast implant rupture. Current versions of STIR incorporate an echo train in order to dramatically shorten acquisition time. Performed as a breathhold scan, this technique has achieved clinical utility in liver imaging.

15.4.2 T2-Weighted Techniques

Standard Multiecho Spin Echo. Standard multiecho spin echo techniques are used when subtle differences in T2 between normal and diseased tissue are expected. A long *TR* (greater than 2000 ms at 1.0 and 1.5 T) is used to minimize T1 saturation of most tissues, though CSF and other fluids are significantly suppressed in signal due to saturation. A short *TE* (less than 20 msec) is used to produce proton-density weighted images while a long *TE* (80 msec or greater) generates T2-weighted images. Gradient motion rephasing is used on the long *TE* image in brain and spine imaging to minimize motion artifacts from bright CSF.

Echo Train Spin Echo. ETSE techniques are useful when high spatial resolution or decreased imaging time is desired for T2-weighted images (e.g., brain, spine, or pelvic imaging). These sequences are best used when T2 differences between normal and diseased tissues are significant since they result in averaging of T2 information. Very long *TR* (greater than 3500 ms) are used to allow coverage of anatomical regions and reduce the amount of signal loss from CSF saturation. Caution should be employed when imaging the liver, particularly in the investigation for hepatocellular carcinoma, because the T2 difference from normal liver may be slight.

Fat Saturation. Fat-suppressed T2-weighted spin echo is useful for liver imaging. Use of this technique results in a decreased phase artifact, expanded dynamic range of tissue signal intensities, and increased conspicuity for focal lesions. It is an excellent technique for imaging capsular-based disease (e.g., hepatosplenic candidiasis or metastases spread through peritoneal seeding) since chemical shift artifacts are absent. Fat saturation can also be applied to echo train and single shot echo train sequences. It is essential to use fat saturation when performing ETSE sequences of the liver to attenuate the signal of fat in the setting of fatty liver, because the high signal of fatty liver on nonsuppressed T2-weighted ETSE sequences can mask the presence of liver lesions. The use of fat suppression on T2-weighted sequences also facilitates the detection of lymph nodes, which appear relatively bright against a background of low signal from suppressed fat.

15.4.3   Sedated or Agitated Patients

Optimal MR imaging results require cooperation from patients to minimize motion artifacts. For brain, spine, or musculoskeletal imaging, pads or restraints may be used to restrict patient movement. For abdominal imaging, patients who are unable to hold their breath because of sedation or decreased consciousness cannot be imaged with breathhold imaging. Spin echo sequences may produce images of good quality. For dynamic scanning following gadolinium-chelate contrast administration, images can be obtained using slice selective 180° inversion pulse prepared snapshot gradient echo sequences (e.g., slice selective Turbo-FLASH, IR-prepared GRASS) followed by either regular or fat-suppressed T1-weighted spin echo techniques.

Patients who are unable to hold their breath or who are slightly agitated require imaging using rapid techniques that are motion insensitive. These include snapshot inversion pulse prepared gradient echo sequences for T1-weighted images and snapshot ETSE for T2-weighted images. These techniques are less sensitive to respiratory motion and acceptable image quality may be obtained.

References and Suggested Readings

Achten, Eric, Paul Boon, Tom Van De Kerchove, Jacques Caemaert, Jacques De Reuek, and Marc Kunnen. 1997. Value of Single-Voxel Proton MR Spectroscopy in Temporal Lobe Epilepsy. *AJNR: American Journal of Neuroradiology* **18,** 1131–1139.

Brown, Mark A., and Richard C. Semelka. 1999. Magnetic Resonance Abbreviations, Definitions, and Descriptions—A Review. *Radiology* (in press).

Chien, Daisy, and Robert R. Edelman. 1991. Ultrafast Imaging Using Gradient Echoes. *Magnetic Resonance Quarterly* **7,** 31–56.

Debatin, Jörg F., and Graeme C. McKinnon, eds. 1998. *Ultrafast MRI: Techniques and Applications.* Springer-Verlag, Heidelberg.

DeYoe, Edgar A., Pater Bandettini, Jay Neitz, David Miller, and Paula Winans. 1994. Functional magnetic resonance imaging (FMRI) of the human brain. *Journal of Neuroscience Methods* **54,** 171–187.

Edelman, Robert R., and Wei Li. 1994. Contrast-enhanced Echo-planar MR Imaging of Myocardial Perfusion: Preliminary Study in Humans. *Radiology* **190,** 771–777.

Edelman, Robert R., Piotr Wielopolski, and Franz Schmitt. 1994. Echo Planar MR Imaging. *Radiology* **192,** 600–612.

Finelli, Daniel A., and Benjamin Kaufman. 1993. Varied Microcirculation of Pituitary Adenomas at Rapid, Dynamic Contrast-Enhanced MR Imaging. *Radiology* **189,** 205–210.

Guyton, Arthur C. 1986. *Textbook of Medical Physiology, 7th ed.* W. B. Saunders, Philadelphia.

Henkelman, R. Mark, and Michael J. Bronskill. 1987. Artifacts in Magnetic Resonance Imaging. *Reviews in Magnetic Resonance Imaging* **2,** 1–126.

Hulka, Carol A., Barbara L. Smith, Dennis C. Sgroi, et al. 1995. Benign and Malignant Breast Lesions: Differentiation with Echo-Planar MR Imaging. *Radiology* **197,** 33–38.

Le Bihan, Denis, ed. 1995. *Diffusion and Perfusion Magnetic Resonance Imaging: Applications to Functional MRI.* Raven Press, New York.

MacFall, James R., H. Cecil Charles, Robert D. Black, et al. 1996. Human Lung Air Spaces: Potential for MR Imaging with Hyperpolarized He-3. *Radiology* **200,** 553–558.

Marks, Michael P., Alex de Crespigny, Daniel Lentz, Dieter R. Enzmann, Gregory W. Albers, and Michael E. Moseley. 1996. Acute and Chronic Stroke: Navigated Spin-Echo Diffusion-Weighted MR Imaging. *Radiology* **199,** 403–408.

Mills, Ian, ed. 1989. *Quantities, Units, and Symbols in Physical Chemistry.* International Union of Pure and Applied Chemistry, Physical Chemistry Division. Blackwell, Oxford, UK.

Mugler, John P., III, and James R. Brookeman. 1988. The Optimum Data Sampling Period for Maximum Signal-to-Noise Ratio in MR Imaging. *Reviews in Magnetic Resonance Imaging* **3,** 1–51.

Mugler, John P., III, Bastiaan Driehuys, James R. Brookeman, et al. 1997. MR Imaging and Spectroscopy Using Hyperpolarized ^{129}Xe Gas: Preliminary Human Results. *Magnetic Resonance in Medicine* **37,** 809–815.

Mukherji, Suresh K., ed. 1998. *Clinical Applications of MR Spectroscopy.* Wiley-Liss, New York.

Parker, Dennis L., and Grant Guilberg. 1990. Signal-to-Noise Efficiency in Magnetic Resonance Imaging. *Medical Physics* **17,** 250–257.

Pipe, J. G., and T. L. Chenevert. 1991. A Progressive Gradient Moment Nulling Design Technique. *Magnetic Resonance in Medicine* **19,** 175–179.

Neil, Jeffrey J. 1997. Measurement of Water Motion (Apparent Diffusion) in Biological Systems. *Concepts in Magnetic Resonance* **9,** 385–401.

Salibi, Nouha, and Mark A. Brown. 1998. *Clinical MR Spectroscopy: First Principles.* Wiley-Liss, New York.

Semelka, Richard C., Susan M. Ascher, and Caroline Reinhold. 1997. *MRI of the Abdomen and Pelvis: A Text Atlas.* Wiley-Liss, New York.

Shaw, D. 1984. *Fourier Transform N.M.R. Spectroscopy, 2nd edition.* Elsevier, Amsterdam, Netherlands.

Shellock, Frank G. 1998. *Pocket Guide to MR Procedures and Metallic Objects: Update 1998.* Lippincott-Raven, Philadelphia.

Slichter, Charles P. 1996. *Principles of Magnetic Resonance, 3rd edition.* Springer-Verlag, Heidelberg.

Stejskal, E. O., and J. E. Tanner. 1963. Spin Diffusion Measurements: Spin Echoes in the Presence of a Time-Dependent Field Gradient. *Journal of Chemical Physics* **42,** 288.

Tannús, Alberto, and Michael Garwood. 1997. Adiabatic Pulses. *NMR in Biomedicine* **10,** 423–434.

Wolff, Steven D., and Robert S. Balaban. 1994. Magnetization Transfer Imaging: Practical Aspects and Clinical Applications. *Radiology* **192,** 593–599.